Expanded Dengue Syndrome

Tauqeer Hussain Mallhi • Yusra Habib Khan
Azreen Syazril Adnan • Nida Tanveer
Raja Ahsan Aftab

Expanded Dengue Syndrome

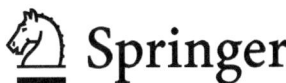 Springer

Tauqeer Hussain Mallhi
Department of Clinical Pharmacy
College of Pharmacy; Jouf University
Sakaka
Saudi Arabia

Azreen Syazril Adnan
Management Science University
Medical Centre
University Drive, Off Persiaran Olahraga
Selangor
Malaysia

Chronic Kidney Disease Resource Centre
School of Medical Sciences
Universiti Sains Malaysia
Kelantan
Malaysia

Raja Ahsan Aftab
Faculty of Health and Medical Sciences
Taylor's University
Selangor
Malaysia

Yusra Habib Khan
Department of Clinical Pharmacy
College of Pharmacy, Jouf University
Sakaka
Saudi Arabia

Nida Tanveer
Jaranwala of Primary and Secondary Health
Care Department
District Headquarter Hospital
Punjab
Pakistan

ISBN 978-981-15-7336-1   ISBN 978-981-15-7337-8   (eBook)
https://doi.org/10.1007/978-981-15-7337-8

This Springer imprint is published by the registered company Springer Nature Singapore Pte Ltd.
The registered company address is: 152 Beach Road, #21-01/04 Gateway East, Singapore 189721, Singapore

Contents

8.3.3   Diagnosis of Dengue-Induced Lymphadenopathy......... 118
8.3.4   Management of Dengue-Induced Lymphadenopathy 118
8.4   Dengue-Induced Splenomegaly............................. 119
8.4.1   Pathogenesis of Dengue-Induced Splenomegaly.......... 119
8.4.2   Clinical Manifestations of Dengue-Induced
Splenomegaly...................................... 119
8.4.3   Diagnosis of Dengue-Induced Splenomegaly 119
8.4.4   Management of Splenomegaly 120
8.5   Dengue-Induced Lymph Node Infarction 120
8.6   Clinical Implications for Healthcare Professionals 121
References.. 121

9   Dengue-Induced Ocular Complications 125
9.1   Ocular Involvements in Dengue Infection..................... 125
9.2   Predictors of Dengue-Related Eye Disease 125
9.3   Common Ocular Symptoms in Dengue Infection 126
9.4   Spectrum of Dengue-Induced Ophthalmic Complications 126
9.4.1   Dengue-Induced Anterior Segment Complications........ 126
9.4.2   Dengue-Induced Posterior Segment Complications 128
9.5   Pathogenesis of Dengue-Induced Ophthalmic Complications...... 131
9.6   Diagnosis of Spectrum of Dengue-Induced Ophthalmic
Complications 132
9.7   Management of Dengue-Induced Ophthalmic Complications 133
9.7.1   Corticosteroids.................................... 133
9.7.2   Intravenous Immunoglobulin (IVIG).................. 134
9.7.3   Other Interventions for Dengue Eye Diseases............ 134
9.8   Prognosis of Dengue Eye Disease 135
References.. 135

10   Dengue-Induced Miscellaneous Complications 137
10.1   Miscellaneous Complications in Dengue Infection............. 137
10.2   Cutaneous Complications in Dengue Infection 137
10.3   Dengue-Induced Skin Rash 138
10.3.1   Hemorrhagic Manifestations of the Skin 139
10.3.2   Differential Diagnosis of Dengue-Induced Skin Rash.... 139
10.3.3   Pathogenesis of Skin Rash......................... 139
10.3.4   Prognosis of Dengue-Induced Skin Rash............... 142
10.4   Oral Complications in Dengue Infection..................... 142
10.4.1   Dengue-Induced Petechiae.......................... 142
10.4.2   Dengue-Induced Epistaxis 143
10.5   Dengue-Induced Intracranial Hemorrhage 143
10.6   Dengue-Induced Thyroiditis 145
10.7   Dengue-Induced Splenial Lesion Syndrome 145
10.8   Dengue-Induced Hemophagocytic Lymphohistiocytosis 146
References.. 147

About the Authors

Tauqeer Hussain Mallhi holds doctoral degree in clinical pharmacy from Universiti Sains Malaysia (USM), Malaysia. Currently, he is working as Assistant Professor in the Department of Clinical Pharmacy, College of Pharmacy at Jouf University (JU), Kingdom of Saudi Arabia since 2019. Previously, he has served as Assistant Professor and Coordinator of the Department of Pharmacy Practice at GC University, Faisalabad, Pakistan. He has also worked as a researcher officer in Chronic Kidney Disease (CKD) Resource Center, Hospital Universiti Sains Malaysia (HUSM), Malaysia. His work broadly concentrates on the epidemiology of dengue infection and explores the burden of acute kidney injury (AKI) and subsequent renal recovery among dengue patients surviving an episode of AKI. He has published more than 70 articles in internationally recognized and peer-reviewed ISI-indexed journals. He has also published 17 book chapters with international publishers. He is currently working on various individual and collaborative research projects including one funded project by the Higher Education Commission (HEC) of Pakistan. He has supervised many master's and PhD students. He is also serving as editorial board member of various peer-reviewed journals related to infectious diseases and health care. Currently, he is investigating atypical manifestations during the course of infectious diseases, with emphasis on renal intricacies. His research work is cutting-edge and worthy of extension in countries where dengue viral infection is endemic. This assertion is in part based on his intensive study of atypical manifestations during dengue infection, which could play a pivotal role in the management of dengue patients. Based on his significant scientific contributions in the field of infectious diseases and nephrology, he has been awarded "Best Presenter Award" and "Best Researcher Award" by the Malaysian Society of Nephrology (MSN) in 2014 and 2017.

Yusra Habib Khan holds master's and doctoral degree in Clinical Pharmacy from Universiti Sains Malaysia (USM), Malaysia. Currently, she is working as Assistant Professor in the Department of Clinical Pharmacy, College of Pharmacy at Jouf University (JU), Kingdom of Saudi Arabia, since 2019. Previously, she has served as Assistant Professor in the Institute of Pharmacy Practice at the Lahore College for Women University, Pakistan. She has also worked as a researcher officer in Chronic Kidney Disease (CKD) Resource Center, Hospital Universiti Sains

Malaysia (HUSM), Malaysia. Her research areas primarily extend to the management of chronic kidney disease (CKD), implications of bioimpedance analysis in nephrology and dengue infection, epidemiology of dengue infection, atypical complications of infectious diseases, and health-related quality of life. She did excellent work on exploring the potential role of bioimpedance analysis in rational use of drugs. She has published more than 75 articles in internationally recognized and peer-reviewed ISI-indexed journals. She has also published 15 book chapters with international publishers. Currently, she is working on various individual and collaborative research projects. Dr Khan has successfully completed project funded by the Higher Education Commission (HEC) of Pakistan and findings have been published in ISI-indexed journal, and she has supervised many postgraduates. She is also serving as an editorial board member of various peer-reviewed journals related to endocrinology, infectious diseases, and nephrology. Currently, she is investigating the utilities and implications of bioimpedance analysis for various infectious diseases. Based on her significant scientific contributions in the field of nephrology, she has been awarded "Best Researcher Award" in 2015 and 2016 by the Universiti Sains Malaysia, Malaysia.

Azreen Syazril Adnan, MD, MMED, FASN is professor of internal medicine and nephrology. He served as the head of Chronic Kidney Disease (CKD) Resource Center and Hemodialysis Unit at Hospital Universiti Sains Malaysia. Currently, he is serving as Consultant Nephrologist and Physician in Management Science University Medical Centre, Malaysia. His research areas include nephrology, infectious nephropathies, tropical infections, and hemodialysis. He has published more than 50 articles in peer-reviewed journals and has delivered numerous plenary presentations in various international meetings. Dr Adnan has supervised many PhD and master's students in the field of nephrology, internal medicine, and pharmaceutical sciences. He is also working as a project leader and team member of several national research projects in Malaysia.

Nida Tanveer, MBBS has graduated from Punjab Medical College Faisalabad, (currently known as Faisalabad Medical University), Pakistan. She is currently working as Women Medical Officer (WMO) in District Headquarter Hospital Jaranwala, Pakistan. Previously, she has served as WMO at various community hospitals including Tehsil Headquarter Hospital (THQ) Chak Jhumra and Rural Health Center (RHC) Chiniot. She has also severed as house officer in Intensive Care Unit (ICU) at Allied Hospital Faisalabad. Her research areas extend to critical care, internal medicine, and infectious diseases. She has published several articles in peer-reviewed journals. Dr Nida is also working on several projects on vector-borne diseases in Pakistan. She has been awarded with several distinguished awards during her career.

Raja Ahsan Aftab holds master's and PhD degrees in clinical pharmacy and is currently working as a Lecturer at Taylor's University, Malaysia. His research areas revolve around clinical trials, chronic disease management, infectious diseases, and health care system development, evaluation, and implementation. He has served as research coordinator at Chronic Kidney Resource Center, Hospital Universiti Sains Malaysia. His research is well acknowledged in various national and international conferences. He has published more than 50 scholarly manuscripts in well-reputed peer-reviewed journals. Dr Aftab is currently supervising postgraduate students and is also a principal investigator for Taylor's University emerging researcher grant scheme.

Dengue Viral Infection (DVI) and Expanded Dengue Syndrome (EDS)

1

1.1   Dengue Viral Infection

Dengue viral infection (DVI) is a debilitating arthropod-borne disease that has been rapidly spread in several regions of the world in recent years [1]. The disease is widespread throughout the tropics, with local variations in risk, and is influenced by rainfall, temperature, and unplanned rapid urbanization. The spectrum of disease varies from mild self-limiting illness to dengue fever (DF) to more severe and fulminating forms, i.e., dengue hemorrhagic fever (DHF) and dengue shock syndrome (DSS) [2, 3].

1.2   Dengue Virus, Vector, and Host

Dengue infection is believed to be caused by dengue virus (DENV), a mosquito-borne single positive stranded RNA virus (family: *Flaviviridae*, genus *Flavivirus*). There are four related but antigenically distinct serotypes of dengue virus designated as DENV-1, DENV-2, DENV-3, and DENV-4 [4]. These four serotypes are genetically similar and share approximately 65% of their genomes [5]. However, a fifth serotype (DENV-5) has been detected during the screening of viral samples in Sarawak state of Malaysia [6]. Dengue virus is transmitted to nonhuman primates (sylvatic form) and humans (human form) via a mosquito vector, primarily of the genus *Aedes* (subgenus: *Stegomyia*). The two most prominent species responsible for DENV transmission are *Aedes aegypti* (origin: Africa) and *Aedes albopictus* (origin: Asia) [7]. The first infection by one serotype produces lifelong, serotype-specific immunity but not lasting protection against infection by another serotype.

This chapter is the part of PhD thesis of Dr. Tauqeer Hussain Mallhi, submitted to the Turnitin repository of Universiti Sains Malaysia

© Springer Nature Singapore Pte Ltd. 2021
T. H. Mallhi et al., *Expanded Dengue Syndrome*,
https://doi.org/10.1007/978-981-15-7337-8_1

Humans are the main amplifying host of the virus that is transmitted to them by the bite of an infective mosquito. The virus undergoes an intrinsic incubation period (IIP—time taken by the virus to complete its development in humans/animals) of 3–14 days (average, 4–7 days), after which the person may experience acute onset of fever accompanied by a variety of nonspecific signs and symptoms. During this acute febrile period (2–10 days), dengue viruses may circulate in the peripheral blood. This human febrile viremic phase (2 days before and 4–5 days after onset of fever) is a source of viruses for other mosquitoes. Dengue virus circulating in the blood of viremic humans is ingested by female mosquitoes during feeding. The virus then infects the mosquito mid-gut and subsequently spreads systemically over a period of 8–12 days. After this extrinsic incubation period (EIP—time taken by the virus to complete its development in mosquitos), the virus can be transmitted to other humans during subsequent probing or feeding. The EIP is influenced in part by environmental conditions, especially ambient temperature. Thereafter the mosquito remains infective for the rest of its life [8]. Figure 1.1 illustrates the cycle of IIP and EIP.

Aedes aegypti is a small, dark mosquito that can be identified by the white bands on its legs and white lyre-shaped markings on its body. It is highly resilient with the ability to rapidly bounce back to initial numbers after disturbances caused by the

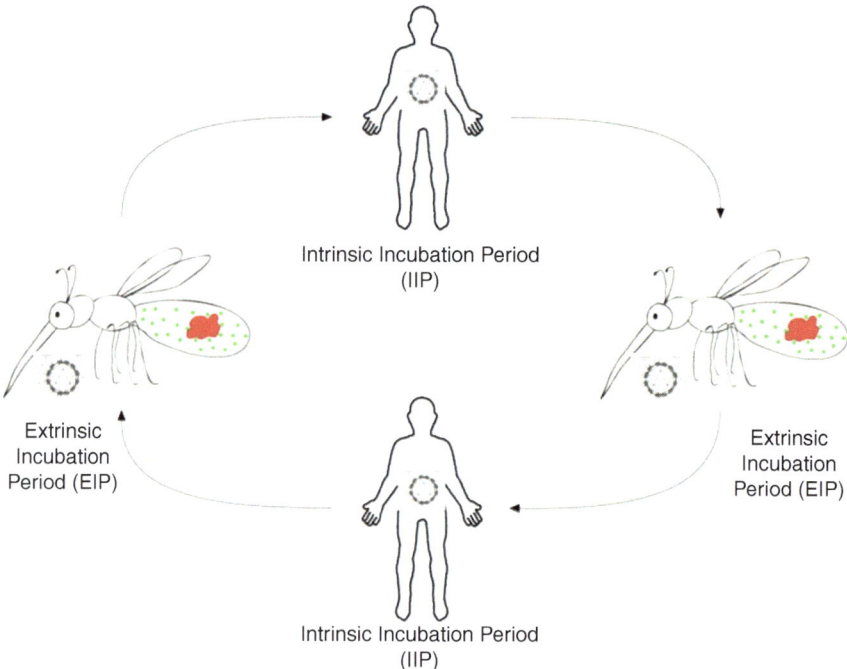

Fig. 1.1 Intrinsic inubation period (host) and extrinsic incubation period (mosquito)—figure is self-constructed

natural disaster or human interventions. *Aedes albopictus*, also known as Asian tiger mosquito, is also a small, dark mosquito with a white dorsal stripes and banded legs. Since *Aedes albopictus* can feed on both human and animals, its survival conditions are more favorable than *Aedes aegypti* [9]. Both vectors differ characteristically from each other [10, 11]. Table 1.1 describes important differences between these two vectors.

1.2.1   Transmission of Dengue Virus

The transmission of DENV occurs in three cycles including enzootic (a primitive sylvatic cycle by monkeys-*Aedes*-monkeys), epizootic (crosses over to nonhuman primates from adjoining human epidemic cycles), and epidemic cycle (human-*Aedes*-human). After ingestion of blood from human, virus replicates in epithelial cell lining of mid-gut and infects the salivary glands. Afterwards, infectious saliva transmits to human primates during probing. DENV also infect genital tract and may enter to fully developed eggs [12]. Dengue transmission usually occurs during rainy season when temperature and humidity are more suitable for breeding of vectors, while in regions where rainfall is scanty, vector breeds in manmade storage containers. However, during dry season, the life cycle of *Aedes aegypti* accelerates, which ultimately results in small-size mosquitos and shorter EIP. Small-size females are required to take more blood meals as protein is needed for egg production; thereby this increases the number of bites and hence infected individuals. Urbanization and increased global travels are some other factors promoting vector breed, thus resulting in higher transmission rates [13].

Table 1.1   Characteristics of two major species of *Aedes* vector

Aedes aegypti	*Aedes albopictus*
• *Origin*: Africa	• *Origin*: Asia
• Highly domesticated	• Maintain feral moorings
• Strong anthropophilic[a]	• Feeds on both human and animals
• Nervous feeder[b]	• Aggressive feeder[c]
• Discordant species[d]	• Concordant species[e]
• High vectorial competency	• High vectorial competency
• Strong vectorial capacity in urban areas while poor in rural regions	• Poor vectorial capacity in urban areas while strong in rural regions

[a]Prefer human beings over animals
[b]Bite more than one host to complete one blood meal
[c]Complete blood meal in one person in one go
[d]Need more than one meal for completion of gonotrophic cycle
[e]Does not require second blood meal for completion of gonotrophic cycle

1.3   Clinical Course of Dengue Infection

After the incubation period, the illness often begins abruptly with fever and follows three phases including febrile, critical, and recovery phase (Fig. 1.2) [10, 11, 15]. The hallmark features of febrile phase include onset of symptoms along with viremia-derived high-grade fever (Table 1.2). Critical phase, also termed as plasma leak phase, is characterized by sudden onset of varying degrees of plasma leak into the pleural and abdominal cavities (Table 1.3). Recovery phase, also referred to as convalescence or reabsorption phase, is a sudden arrest of plasma leak with concomitant reabsorption of extravasated plasma and fluids (Table 1.4) [15].

All the three phases of clinical course of dengue infection are characterized by specific clinico-laboratory features and serology and virology pattern [10, 11]. Summary of the clinical course of DVI is presented in Fig. 1.3 [27, 28].

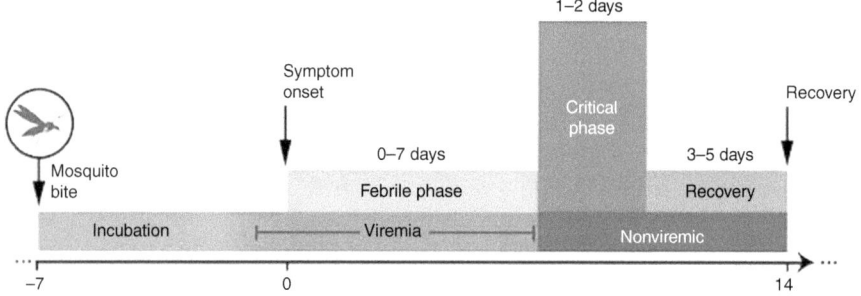

Fig. 1.2 Three phases during the clinical course of dengue infection (This figure is adapted and modified from the website of the Centers for Disease Control and Prevention [14]. Figure is not copyright protected)

Table 1.2 Recovery phase of dengue viral infection

Characteristics	Typical duration for this phase ranges from 0 to 7 days and biphasic fever can occur. Monitoring of defervescence (may occur between 3 and 8 days of illness) and warning signs is crucial to identify progression to critical phase [15]
Clinical manifestations	This phase is often accompanied by onset of high temperature accompanied by severe headache, retro-orbital pain, myalgia, arthralgia, transient macular or maculopapular rash, facial flushing or erythema, injected oropharynx, nausea, vomiting, anorexia, and minor hemorrhagic manifestations such as petechia, ecchymosis, purpura, epistaxis, gum bleeding, hematuria, vaginal and gastrointestinal bleeding, or positive tourniquet test. The liver may be large or tender after few days of fever. Onset of fever may also cause limited daily activity [16]
Laboratory findings	Leucopenia, mild to moderate thrombocytopenia, hyponatremia, and elevated aspartate aminotransferase [17] and alanine aminotransferase (ALT) can occur during this phase [18]
Complications	Febrile phase may cause several complications such as dehydration, hyponatremia, seizures in young children (due to fever), and neurological manifestations (encephalitis and aseptic meningitis) [19, 20]

Table 1.3 Critical phase of dengue viral infection

Characteristics	This phase typically starts around the time of defervescence; however, it may begin early among patients who are febrile on the third day of onset of fever and lasts about 24–48 h. During the febrile to afebrile transition, patients without increased capillary permeability improve and do not go through the critical phase. On the other hand, patients with increased capillary permeability may manifest with the warning signs, primarily due to plasma leakage. Onset of critical phase can be identified by rapid decline in platelet (PLT) count with a concomitant rise in hematocrit (HCT) and presence of warning signs. Moreover, patients may develop leucopenia up to 24 h before platelet drop is recognized [21]. The presence of warning signs indicates the beginning of critical phase. Therefore, the following warning signs should be observed before or at the time of defervescence during dengue infection [11] • Clinical fluid accumulation (ascites, pleural effusion) • Liver enlargement > 2 cm • Severe abdominal pain or tenderness • Persistent vomiting (at least 3 episodes/24 h) • Mucosal bleed • Lethargy or restlessness • Sometimes rapid decline in PLT count with concurrent increase hematocrit in (HCT) is also considered warning sign
Clinical manifestations	Progressive leukopenia followed by a rapid reduction in PLT count and increased HCT above baseline usually precedes plasma leakage. The degree of plasma leakage varies and usually reflects with the degree of hemoconcentration (as determined by elevated HCT). However, degree of hemoconcentration is affected by intravenous fluid (IVF) therapy. An early IV therapy can reduce hemoconcentration; therefore, frequent monitoring of HCT levels is essential for the adjustment of IVF therapy. Pleural effusion and ascites are mostly clinically detectable after IVF therapy only, unless plasma leakage is significant. In addition to the plasma leakage, hemorrhagic manifestations such as easy bruising and bleeding at venipuncture sites occur frequently [21] In most of the cases with plasma leakage, circulatory changes are minimal or transient, and many of patients recover spontaneously or after fluid/electrolyte therapy. However, patients with severe plasma leakage may develop shock due to loss of critical plasma volume. With profound and/or prolonged shock, hypoperfusion results in metabolic acidosis, progressive organ impairment, and disseminated intravascular coagulation (DIVC) which leads to severe hemorrhage, causing reduced HCT in severe shock. Instead of the leukopenia usually seen during this phase of dengue, the total white cell count (WBCs) may increase as a stress response to severe bleeding. In addition, severe organ involvement may develop. Some patients progress to the critical phase of plasma leakage and shock before defervescence [10, 11]
Laboratory findings	Critical phase causes marked disturbances in laboratory parameters that include increased HCT (hemoconcentration), moderate to severe thrombocytopenia, leukopenia, and transient increase in activated partial thromboplastin time (aPTT) with decrease in fibrinogen [22]
Complications	Hypovolemic shock from plasma leakage, end-organ impairment due to prolonged shock, severe hemorrhage, and encephalopathy are some major complications during critical phase [10]

Table 1.4 Recovery phase of dengue viral infection (DVI)

Characteristics	If the patient survives critical phase, a gradual reabsorption of extravascular fluid in the next 48–72 h occurs. However, recovery depends on the severity of illness and treatments provided during febrile and critical phase [23]
Clinical manifestations	Clinical clues of recovery phase include patient's improvement, hemodynamic stability, severe fatigue, and increased diuresis. Moreover, second rash that might be macular or erythematous with small circular islands of normal, unaffected skin may appear. This convalescent rash can be very pruritic and desquamate. Bradycardia and electrocardiographic changes are common during this stage [24]
Laboratory findings	Stable HCT or slightly elevated due to dilutional effect of reabsorbed plasma (hemodilution), rise in WBCs soon after defervescence, increase PLT after WBC recovery [22]
Complications	Respiratory distress may occur from massive pleural effusion and ascites. Hypervolemia, congestive heart failure (CHF), and acute pulmonary edema can occur if IVF therapy has been provided excessively or if it is extended for long duration. Organ impairment can result due to prolonged or refractory shock. This might include ischemic hepatitis and hepatic encephalopathy. Nosocomial infections can occur, especially in infants and elderly patients [25]

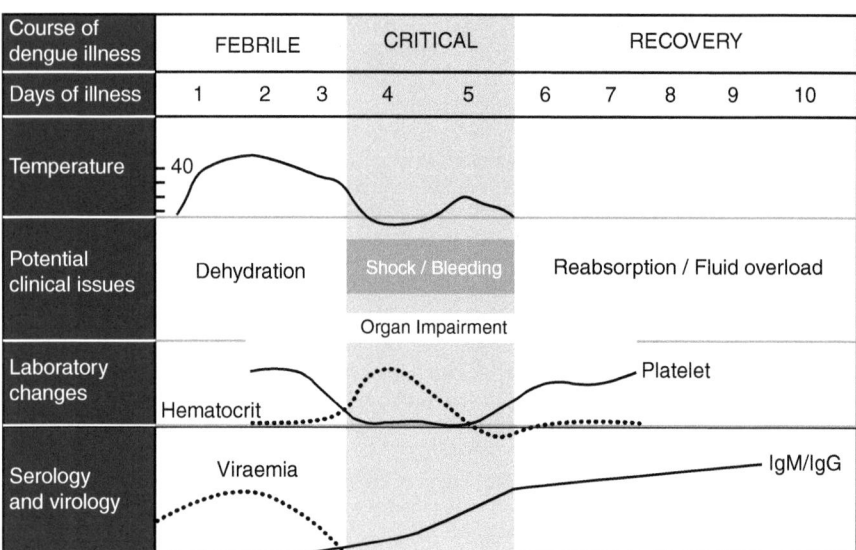

Fig. 1.3 Summary of the clinical course of dengue infection (Descriptive note: Figure is reprinted from reference [26] and has no copyright restrictions)

1.4   Diagnosis of Dengue Infection

Dengue can be diagnosed either by isolation of virus or by serological and molecular methods. Early and accurate diagnosis of DVI is of paramount importance for surveillance, management, research, and detection of circulating serotypes.

Table 1.5 Types of diagnostic tests for dengue infection

Technique	Recommended time, specificity, and sensitivity
Antibody detection	
IgM detection	4 days after onset of symptoms and up to 3 months in primary dengue 3 days after onset of symptoms and sometimes hindered by large-scale IgG production in secondary dengue (Sensitivity, 61.5–100%; specificity, 52–100%)
IgG detection	10 days after onset of symptom in primary dengue 3 days after onset of symptoms in secondary dengue (Sensitivity, 46.4–99%; specificity, 80–100%)
Rapid IgM detection (strips)	5 days after onset of symptoms and up to 2 months (Sensitivity, 20.5–97.7%; specificity, 76.6–96.6%)
Antigen/antibody combined detection	
NS1 and IgM combo kit	As this is a combo test, useful in early stage of infection (day 3 onwards) and up to sero-conversion period (up to 2 weeks onwards) (Sensitivity, 89.9–92.9%; specificity, 75–100%)
NS1 and IgM/IgG combo kit	As this is a combo test, useful in early stage of infection (day 3 onwards) and up to sero-conversion period (up to 2 weeks onwards). In the event of both NS1 and IgM are non-reactive and IgG is reactive, case can be interpreted as secondary dengue. (Sensitivity, 93%; specificity, 100%)
Viral detection	
Virus isolation (cell culture)	1–5 days of onset of symptoms in primary dengue and 1–4 days after onset of symptoms in secondary dengue (sensitivity, 40.5%; specificity, 100%)
Virus isolation (mosquitoes)	Same as above (sensitivity, 71.5–84.2%; specificity, 100%)
Viral RNA RT-PCR (conventional)	Same as above (sensitivity, 48.4–100%; specificity, 100%)
Viral RNA RT-PCR (real time)	Same as above (sensitivity, 58.9–100%; specificity, 100%)
Viral antigen (NS1)	1–7 days of onset of symptoms in primary dengue and 1–5 days after onset of symptoms in secondary dengue (sensitivity, 54.2–93.4%; specificity, 92.5–100%)

Abbreviations: *IgM* immunoglobulin M, *IgG* immunoglobulin G, *NS1* non-structural protein 1, *RNA* ribonucleic acid, *RT-PCR* reverse transcriptase polymerase chain reaction
Reference: Information provided in the table is extracted from [26]

Diagnostic tests used to confirm DVI are described in Table 1.5 [26]. The use of diagnostic tests varies among hospitals depending upon the availability and nature of dengue infection. However, diagnostic tests include point-of-care testing such as dengue NS1 antigen test and rapid combo tests (NS1 antigen and dengue IgM/IgG antibodies) [29].

Dengue rapid combo test (NS1 and IgM) or NS1 antigen should be carried out among suspected cases. However, the type of diagnostic test should be based on patient's clinical history [30]. Table 1.6 demonstrates the recommendations of diagnostic tests according to the clinical history of patients.

Table 1.6 Recommendation of type of dengue test based on the clinical history of patients and interpretation of their results

Clinical history (test)	Results	Interpretations
Fever < 5 days (dengue NS1 or RCT)	Positive	Acute dengue infection
	Negative	DVI still cannot rule out. Repeat for dengue IgM after day 5 of fever
Fever > 5 days (dengue IgM)	Positive	Suggestive of recent dengue infection
	Intermediate	Repeat
	Negative	The result does not rule out dengue infection. Repeat sample for dengue IgM after day 7 of fever or dengue IgG test
Fever > 5 days and dengue IgM and/or NS1 was negative (dengue IgG)	Positive	Elevated IgG levels are seen in acute or past infections. A titer of ≥1:2560 is consistent with acute secondary infection
	Intermediate	Repeat if clinically indicated
	Negative	The absence of elevated IgG is presumptive evidence that the patient does not have secondary dengue infection

Abbreviations: *NS1* non-structural protein 1, *RCT* rapid combo test, *DVI* dengue viral infection, *IgM* immunoglobulin M, *IgG* immunoglobulin G
Reference: [26]

1.5   Dengue Case Classification

The World Health Organization (WHO) classified DVI in 1997 as undifferentiated fever, dengue fever (DF), and dengue hemorrhagic fever (DHF), where DHF was further divided into four grades (grades I–IV). Grades III and IV are referred to as dengue shock syndrome (DSS) [31]. Due to complexity and applicability of previous 1997 criteria, WHO has proposed new dengue classification in 2009. According to this new definition, dengue is classified into two types based on its severity: non-severe dengue (dengue with and without warning signs) and severe dengue [11]. However, the older classification is still widely used, as WHO's Regional Office for Southeast Asia (SEARO) has included 1997 definition in its revised and expanded guidelines for DVI [10]. Nevertheless, there has been a considerable debate regarding the value of both 1997 and 2009 classifications [16]. More recently, the Centers of Disease Control and Prevention (CDC) classified DVI into three types, i.e., dengue, dengue-like illness, and severe dengue. Dengue-like illness is defined by fever and included in the list of notifiable infectious conditions [32]. The use of criteria for dengue classification depends on discretion of treating physician and hospital or national dengue guidelines. The details of WHO and WHO/SEARO criteria is given below.

1.5.1 Dengue Case Classification [36]

This classification provides information to identify probable and confirm dengue cases that can further be classified into severe and non-severe dengue infection as demonstrated by Fig. 1.4 [11].

1.5.2 Dengue Case Classification [34]

WHO's Regional Office for Southeast Asia (SEARO) has revised dengue guidelines in 2011 and classified DVI into asymptomatic infection, viral syndrome, dengue fever (DF), and dengue hemorrhagic fever (DHF) including dengue shock syndrome (DSS) (Fig. 1.5). However, the classification used in these contemporary guidelines corresponds to [35] criteria [11].

Grading the severity of the disease has been found clinically and epidemiologically useful in both children and adults [10, 31]. The severity of DHF is classified into four grades (Table 1.7) where presence of thrombocytopenia with concurrent hemoconcentration differentiates grade I and grade II from dengue fever.

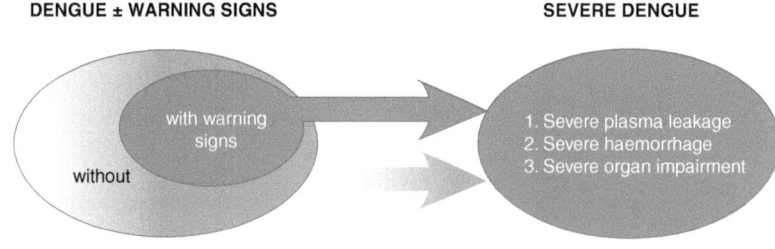

DENGUE ± WARNING SIGNS   **SEVERE DENGUE**

with warning signs

without

1. Severe plasma leakage
2. Severe haemorrhage
3. Severe organ impairment

CRITERIA FOR DENGUE ± WARNING SIGNS

Probable dengue

live in /travel to dengue endemic area.
Fever and 2 of the folbwing criteria:

- Nausea, vomiting
- Rash
- Aches and pains
- Tourniquet test positive
- Leukopenia
- Any warning sign

Laboratory-confirmed dengue
lirrportant when no sign of plasma leakage)

Warning signs*

- Abdominal pain or tenderness
- Persistent vomiting
- Clinical Ruid accumulation
- Mucosal bleed
- Lethargy, resdessness
- Uver enlargment >2 em
- Laboratory: increase in HCT concurrent with rapid decrease in platelet count

*Ireqtiring strict observation and medical interverlion)

CRITERIA FOR SEVERE DENGUE

Severe plasma leakage
leading to:

- Shock (DSS)
- Fluid accumulation with respiratory distress

Severe bleeding
as evaluated by dinician

Severe organ involvement
- Liver: AST or ALT >= 1 000
- CNS: Impaired consciousness
- Heart and other organs

Fig. 1.4 WHO 2009 criteria for dengue classification

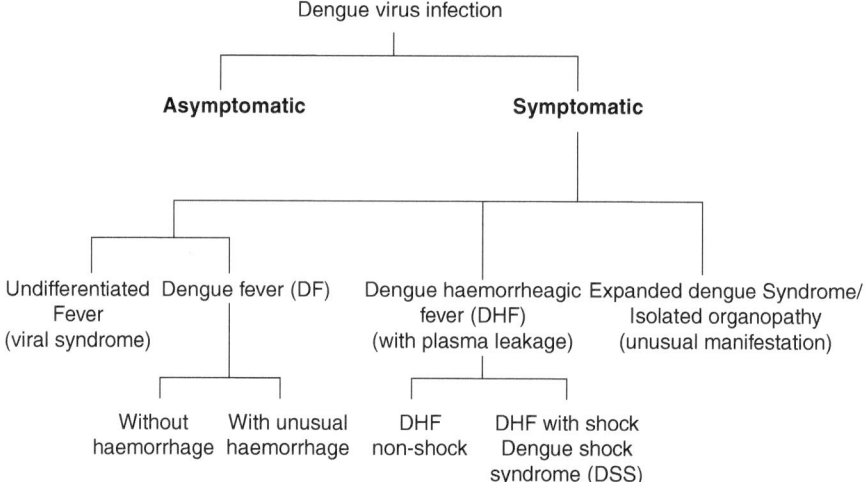

Fig. 1.5 WHO and SEARO 2011 or WHO 1999 criteria for dengue classification (Reference: Figure is adapted from WHO criteria for dengue classification which has no copyright restrictions)

Table 1.7 Classification of dengue viral infection according to WHO and SEARO (2011) and WHO (1997)

DVI classification	Sign and symptoms	Laboratory findings
DF	Fever with two of the following: • Headache • Retro-orbital pain • Myalgia • Arthralgia/bone pain • Rash • Hemorrhagic manifestations • No evidence of plasma leakage	Leucopenia (WBC ≤ 5000 cells/mm^3) Thrombocytopenia (platelet count <150,000 cells/mm^3) Rising hematocrit (5–10%) No evidence of plasma loss
DHF (grade I)	Fever and hemorrhagic manifestation (positive tourniquet test) and evidence of plasma leakage	Thrombocytopenia <100,000 cells/mm3; HCT rise ≥20%
DHF (grade II)	As in grade I plus spontaneous bleeding	Thrombocytopenia <100,000 cells/mm^3; HCT rise ≥20%
DHF (grade III)	As in grade I or II plus circulatory failure (weak pulse, narrow pulse pressure (≤20 mmHg), hypotension, restlessness)	Thrombocytopenia <100,000 cells/mm^3; HCT rise ≥20%
DHF (grade IV)	As in grade III plus profound shock with undetectable BP and pulse	Thrombocytopenia <100,000 cells/mm^3; HCT rise ≥20%

Abbreviations: *DF* dengue fever, *DHF* dengue hemorrhagic fever, *WBC* white blood cells, *HCT* hematocrit
DHF grade III and IV is dengue shock syndrome (DSS)
Reference: [10, 31]

1.6   Global Prevalence and Burden of Dengue Viral Infection

The global burden of dengue is formidable and represents a growing challenge to health authorities. Knowledge of geographical distribution and burden of dengue is essential for understanding its contribution to global morbidity and mortality. It will further help to determine resource allocation to control disease and to evaluate international impact of these control activities [37].

The incidence of dengue has grown dramatically around the world in recent decades. However, the actual numbers of dengue cases are underreported or misclassified. One recent estimate indicates 390 million dengue infections per year, of which 96 million manifests clinically with any severity of disease [37]. Although the exact global burden of the disease is uncertain, the number of WHO reported cases has increased from 2.2 million in 2010 to 3.2 million in 2015. Before 1970, only nine countries had dengue epidemics. Currently, dengue is endemic in more than 100 countries, 5 out of the 6 WHO regions. Today about 40% of world's population live in dengue risk areas. Every year approximately 5 lac people with severe dengue require hospitalization and 2.5% of those affected die [15, 38, 39].

The surge in dengue has been most marked in Asia and accounts 75% of global dengue burden, costing Southeast Asia [11] US$1billion annually. It is estimated that among 2.5 billion people at risk globally, about 1.8 billion reside in Asia. Southeast Asia records approximately 2.9 million dengue episodes and 5906 fatality cases annually, with a yearly monetary burden of $950 million [40]. Recurrent dengue epidemics in Asia have established hyperendemic areas, often in large and heavily populated cities. In Southeast Asia, demands of a large health and economic burden for dengue control are more challenging than ever. The year 2015 was characterized by large dengue outbreaks in Asia, with the Philippines and Malaysia representing 59.5% and 16% increase in case numbers to the previous year, respectively. Alarmingly, spread of *Aedes albopictus* (a secondary dengue vector) from Asia to North America and Europe may result in high disease burden in these cooler temperate regions [41].

1.7   Management of Dengue Viral Infection

Despite myriad improvements in the clinical care of dengue patients, there are no specific antiviral agents to treat the infection. Management of DVI primarily revolves around supportive care with particular emphasis on vigilant fluid administration. The primary aim during the management of dengue infection is to limit the complications and to reduce the severity during the disease course. In this context, fluid therapy in accordance with the disease severity has become primary intervention in dengue management [11]. WHO recommends a stepwise disease management approach for dengue cases as shown in Fig. 1.6.

A careful history of dengue patients is of paramount importance for appropriate diagnosis and treatment. Generally, the diagnosis in many endemic countries is usually a presumptive via clinical evidence of acute febrile illness with decreased

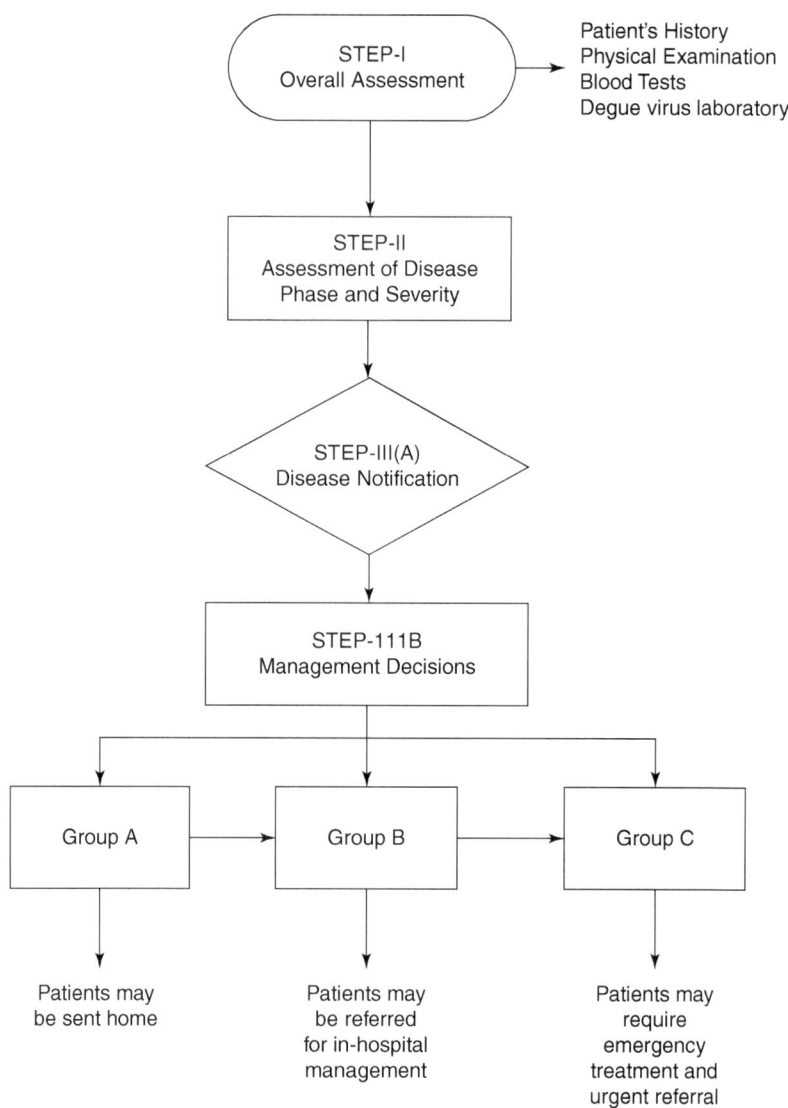

Fig. 1.6 A stepwise approach for the management of dengue infection (Descriptive note: This figure is self-constructed)

platelet count. The tourniquet test is an important basic screening tool for dengue. The WHO also suggests using the tourniquet test as a vital parameter in the diagnosis of dengue [23]. Full blood count should be performed at the first visit. Liver function tests, glucose, serum electrolytes, urinalysis, cardiac enzymes, and electrocardiogram can be performed subjected to their need and availability [42].

1.7.1   Management of Group A Patients

Patients who can tolerate adequate amount of oral fluids, pass urine every 6 h, and have no warning signs are classified as Group A patients. These patients may be sent home with home care instructions including oral fluid therapy and fever management by paracetamol. However, patients or caregivers should be advised to seek hospital care if there are no clinical improvement, presence of warning signs, and absence of urination [43].

1.7.2   Management of Group B Patients

Dengue patients with warnings signs are included in Group B. Moreover, there are certain conditions which can complicate the dengue illness and its management. These conditions include comorbidities (diabetes mellitus, renal failure, obesity, and chronic hemolytic diseases), old age, infancy, and pregnancy. All the patients with one or more of these conditions are also classified in Group B. In addition, patients who are experiencing the social constraints such as living alone or living far from a health facility without reliable means of transport are placed in this group.

1.7.2.1   Management of Group B Patients with Warning Signs

For Group B patients, fluid replacement should be carefully carried out and must be performed under close observation in a hospital. Intravenous fluid replacement by either colloids or crystalloids should be considered in order to prevent shock [44]. A reference hematocrit level must be assessed before initiation of therapy. Isotonic solutions (0.9% saline, Ringer's lactate, or Hartmann's solution) should be started at a dose of 5–7 ml/kg/h for 1–2 h. The dose can be reduced after 2–4 h up to 2–3 ml/kg/h. Water and electrolyte status should be maintained during treatment to avoid under- and over-administration of fluid. If the vital signs are worsening and hematocrit is rapidly increasing, the infusion rate should be increased to 5–10 ml/ kg/h for 1–2 h. It must be noted that the minimum intravenous fluid volume required to maintain adequate perfusion and urine output is 0.5 ml/kg/h. Intravenous fluids are usually needed for only 24–48 h [45]. The parameters which should be monitored for these patients include warning signs, vital signs, peripheral perfusion (1–4 h), urine output (4–6 h), hematocrit (before and after fluid replacement and then 6–12 h), blood glucose, and other organ functions (such as renal profile, liver profile, and coagulation profile). This monitoring should be done for at least 1 day after the discontinuation of intravenous fluid to prevent possible fluid intoxication (due to fluid redistribution) in the convalescent phase [23].

1.7.2.2   Management of Group B Patients Without Warning Signs

These patients are managed in a similar way as Group B patients with warning signs. However, these patients may be able to take oral fluids after a few hours of intravenous fluid therapy. Patients should be monitored for temperature pattern, volume of fluid intake and losses, urine output (volume and frequency), warning signs, hematocrit, and white blood cell and platelet counts. Other laboratory tests (such as liver and renal functions tests) can be performed, depending on the clinical need and the facilities of the hospital [25].

1.7.3   Management of Group C Patients

Dengue patients with severe plasma leakage, fluid accumulation with respiratory distress, severe hemorrhage, and severe organ impairments require hospitalization with access to intensive care facilities and blood transfusion. These patients are classified in Group C, and judicious intravenous fluid resuscitation is the essential and usually sole intervention. Isotonic crystalloid solutions should be the first priority for the patients. Moreover, isotonic colloid solutions should be used among severe patients presenting with profound shock. Colloids can also be used for the patients demonstrating no response to initial crystalloid therapy [46]. The goals of fluid resuscitation include improving central and peripheral circulation (decreasing tachycardia, improving blood pressure, pulse volume, warm and pink extremities, capillary refill time <2 s) and improving end-organ perfusion (stable conscious level, urine output ≥0.5 ml/kg/h, decreasing metabolic acidosis) [24].

1.7.3.1 Management of Compensated Shock

Compensated shock (maintained systolic pressure with evidence of reduced perfusions) can be treated with IV isotonic crystalloids at rate 5–10 ml/kg/h for at least 1 h. If the conditions of patients improve, the dose can be reduced to 5–7 ml/kg/h for 1–2 h, then to 3–5 ml/kg/h for 2–4 h, then to 2–3 ml/kg/h, and further depending on hemodynamic status. For patients with persistent shock (vital signs are still unstable), the levels of hematocrit must be evaluated, and if found high (>50%), repeat second bolus dose at 10–20 ml/kg/h for 1 h. However, caution should be exercised to maintain the fluid therapy for 24–48 h. Hematocrit is the primary monitoring parameter in such patients and it should be monitored every 6–8 h [47].

1.7.3.2 Management of Hypotensive Shock

The management of hypotensive shock is more vigorous than compensated shock. Both crystalloids and colloids can be initiated at 20 ml/kg as a bolus given over 15 min. If the patient's condition improves, infusion rate can be reduced to 10 ml/kg/h for 1 h, then to 5–7 ml/kg/h for 1–2 h, then to 3–5 ml/kg/h for 2–4 h, and finally to 2–3 ml/kg/h or less. The infusion rate should be maintained for up to 24–48 h. For clinically unstable patients, second dose of colloids (for 30–60 min) and blood transfusion should be considered with periodic monitoring of hematocrit levels. Further boluses of the fluids titrated to the clinical response should be given in case of no improvements. Hematocrit and urine output are primary parameters of observation during the treatment of hypotensive shock in patients [23, 25, 48]. Caution must be practiced during IV fluid administration to avoid any drug therapy-related problems. Since development of fluid overload is the major therapy-associated complication, a careful monitoring of parenteral fluid therapy is of utmost importance. Fluid administration should be kept to the minimum required level to maintain cardiovascular stability until permeability reverts to a normal level [15].

1.7.4   Management of Hemorrhagic Complications

Dengue patients presenting with severe bleeding can be managed with blood transfusion. However, it requires careful administration amid the risks of fluid overload. Transfusion of platelet concentrates and/or fresh frozen plasma, fresh-packed red cells, fresh whole blood, and cryoprecipitate at 10 ml/kg may also be needed depending on the coagulation profile. The prophylactic use of platelets is not well established for patients without clinically significant bleeding and even in the presence of marked thrombocytopenia [49, 50]. The prophylactic use of platelet transfusions is increasingly recognized in the dengue-endemic countries. However, this prophylaxis is associated with substantial clinical risks and costs of care. These findings necessitate the dire need of well-controlled clinical trials to establish the role of platelet transfusions as prophylactic measure. In patients with severe dengue infection, adjuvant therapy including vasopressor and inotropic agents, renal replacement therapy, and further treatment of organ impairment may be necessary [50].

1.7.5   Management of Fluid Overload

Fluid overload with large pleural effusions and ascites is a common cause of acute respiratory distress and respiratory failure in severe dengue. The management of fluid overload can be initiated with immediate oxygen therapy preceding discontinuation of IV fluids. Oral or IV furosemide can be recommended to patients depending upon the volume of fluid overload. It must be noted that minimum IV fluid therapy should be carried out to maintain euglycemia among patients [11, 51].

1.7.6   New Treatments for Dengue Infection

The preferable new treatment for dengue would be an antiviral drug. At present, a specific antiviral drug is not available; however, there have been a lot of attempts to discover one. In phytomedicine, several sulfated polysaccharides extracted from seaweeds have been studied, and high antiviral activity against dengue virus has been observed [52]. In modern medicine, ribavirin, glycyrrhizin, and 6-azauridine are reported to have cytostatic and inhibitory effects on the dengue virus [53]. An adenosine analog is another promising drug that is currently being studied. The chemical "NITD008" is an adenosine analog inhibitor that interrupts the RNA-dependent RNA polymerase of flaviviruses [54].

The establishment of a therapeutic pipeline and the design of randomized, controlled trials of drugs targeting the virus or the immune response are recent developments. Recent trials have assessed chloroquine, oral prednisolone, and balapiravir for the treatment of dengue infection. Various trials on statins and other antiviral drugs are in process of planning and execution. However, preliminary results from these trials are not in favor of the use of any specific therapeutic agent for dengue [15, 55].

1.7.7   Vaccines of Dengue Infection

Dengvaxia® is the currently approved vaccine for the prevention of DVI. It is a live recombinant tetravalent vaccine available in several countries and recommended in three doses at 0, 6, and 12 months. Initial findings have demonstrated the risk reduction of severe illness and hospitalization up to 30% among individuals with previous history of dengue infection with one or more DENV strains. However, this vaccine is found to be less effective for individuals without any previous history of infection, particularly those residing in low prevalent regions [56]. It must be noted that vaccine may initiate the dengue infection among people having no previous exposure to the virus and the subsequent infection (secondary infection) with any serotype in these individuals may result in severe disease. In this context, the WHO issued advisory stating that vaccination can be considered as a component of comprehensive dengue control strategy only in the regions having high burden of the disease [57]. Thus, vaccine should possibly be avoided by the countries with low prevalence of infection and must be used with caution in high burden areas, particularly in hyperendemic regions.

The development of vaccine against dengue infection remained slow amid the fact that the immunity to a single DENV can attribute to the severe infection. A clinically effective dengue vaccine should provide high levels of immunity against all four serotypes of dengue virus [58]. However, sero-conversion alone does not predict protection against the infection. Various tetravalent vaccines have been developed and currently under investigations in different phases of clinical trials [59].

1.8   Prevention and Control of Dengue Viral Infection (DVI)

The prevention and control of dengue infections depends largely on preventing factors such as environmental control, biological control, chemical control, and active case surveillance [35].

1.8.1   Environmental Control

Measures should be taken for reducing vector breeding sites, solid waste management, modification of manmade breeding sites, and improvements in house design. For the controls to be effective, public programs should be conducted [60]. Personal protection, household insecticide, natural repellents, and chemical repellents are important to avoid man–vector contact.

1.8.2   Biological Control of the Vector

Larval stages of the dengue vector are main targets in biological control. These include the use of copepod crustaceans, endotoxin-producing bacteria, and larvivorous fish. *Bacillus thuringiensis* serotype H-14 is more effective against *A. aegypti* with very low levels of mammalian toxicity [35].

1.8.3   Chemical Control

Larvicidal pesticides and space spray are used mainly as means of chemical control. Where, space spraying is more readily employed due to financial constraints related to insecticides. Space sprays are usually applied as thermal fogs or ultra-low volume sprays. Both these methods are equally effective; however, thermal fogging is more common. Insecticides containing malathion, fenitrothion, or pirimiphos-methyl are effectively used; however, there are reports of mosquito vector resistance against these insecticides [61, 62].

1.9   Expanded Dengue Syndrome

In recent years with the geographical spread of dengue and more involvement of adults, there have been increasing reports of DVI with unusual manifestations, termed as "expanded dengue syndrome" (EDS). These atypical and unusual organopathies include intricacies of major organs, such as the liver, kidney, heart, lungs, and nervous system, and could be explained as complication of severe profound shock or associated with underlying host conditions or co-infections. The involvements of various organs are increasingly being reported in DHF, while EDS can also occur during DF without any evidence of plasma leakage [10, 38, 39]. These atypical manifestations were previously termed as "unusual complications" by WHO [11, 31]. Currently, EDS is new entity incorporated to WHO guidelines. The immunopathological mechanisms during dengue infection primarily target endothelium, resulting in vascular permeability and coagulation disorders that can explain these varied systemic involvements [63]. The spectrum of EDS is described in Fig. 1.7.

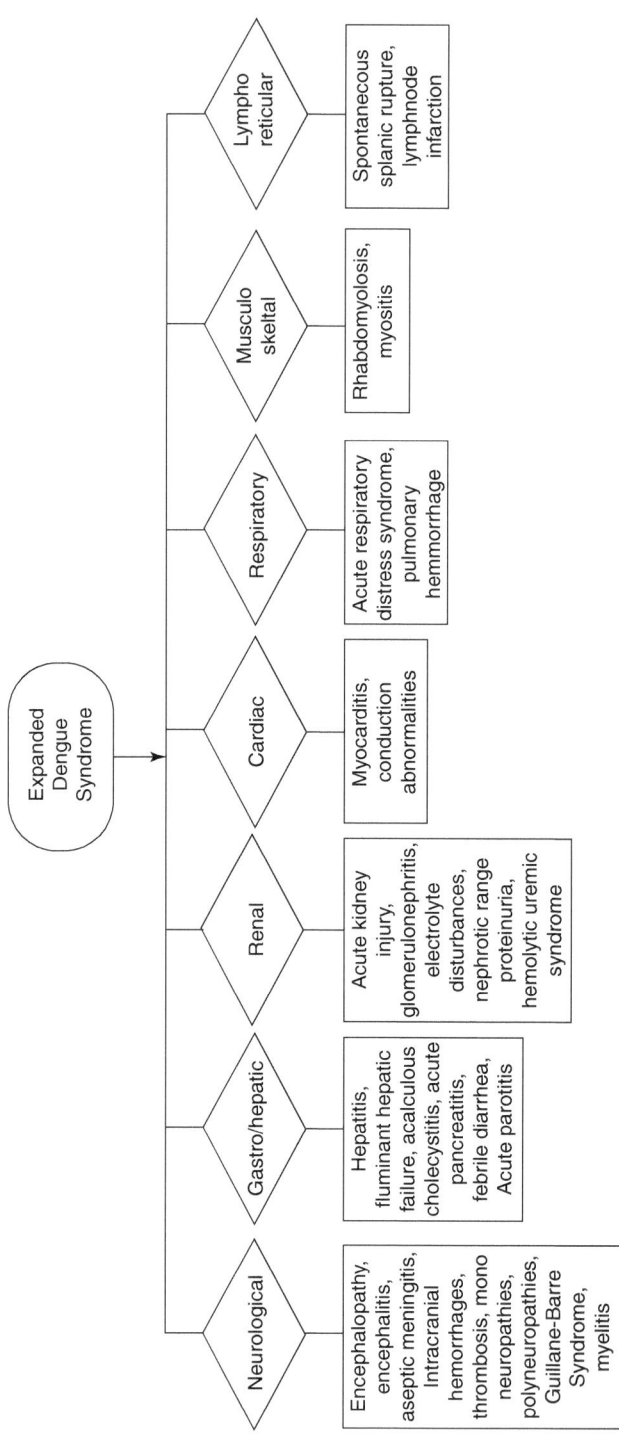

Fig. 1.7 Manifestations of expanded dengue syndrome. Reference: World Health Organization Regional Office for Southeast Asia. Comprehensive guidelines for prevention and control of dengue and dengue hemorrhagic guidelines, 2011 [10]

1.9.1   Pathogenesis of EDS

The pathogenesis of EDS is not clear amid lack of studies on animal models. In the absence of in vitro experiments, disease spectrum is difficult to be elucidated and mimicked for humans [37]. However, autopsy data from human studies is of utmost importance and provide satisfactory answers of various questions related to etiological factors of EDS. These studies also provide information on target tissues and possible mechanisms through which dengue virus can infect the specific organs. Most of these studies report histopathological findings among dengue fatal cases and report the liver, spleen, and lymph nodes as major target organs for dengue virus [64–66]. The liver is the most studied organ during the course of DVI. Recent findings on dengue fatal cases illustrate that hepatic complications are not only limited to hemorrhage and edema in the liver but also extended to other intricacies caused by metabolic alterations and inflammatory reactions. These hepatic complications include steatosis, areas with infiltrated cells, necrosis, hyperplasia, and destruction of Kupffer cells [64, 65, 67]. Moreover, lesions of spleen tissues are widely discussed in the literature. The lesions include but are not limited to interstitial edema, vascular congestion, splenic rupture, and bleeding [64, 65, 67]. Recent advances on research on atypical complications of EDS demonstrate the involvement of other major organs such as the kidney, lung, heart, and central nervous system. Histopathological findings demonstrate the presence of hemorrhage, edema, and inflammatory infiltrates in these organs [3, 17, 63, 68–71].

References

1. Messina JP, Brady OJ, Scott TW, Zou C, Pigott DM, Duda KA, et al. Global spread of dengue virus types: mapping the 70 year history. Trends Microbiol. 2014;22(3):138–46.
2. Deen JL, Harris E, Wills B, Balmaseda A, Hammond SN, Rocha C, et al. The WHO dengue classification and case definitions: time for a reassessment. Lancet. 2006;368(9530):170–3.
3. Mallhi TH, Khan AH, Sarriff A, Adnan AS, Khan YH. Determinants of mortality and prolonged hospital stay among dengue patients attending tertiary care hospital: a cross-sectional retrospective analysis. BMJ Open. 2017;7(7):e016805.
4. Khan NA, Azhar EI, El-Fiky S, Madani HH, Abuljadial MA, Ashshi AM, et al. Clinical profile and outcome of hospitalized patients during first outbreak of dengue in Makkah, Saudi Arabia. Acta Trop. 2008;105(1):39–44.
5. Gubler DJ. Epidemic dengue/dengue hemorrhagic fever as a public health, social and economic problem in the 21st century. Trends Microbiol. 2002;10(2):100–3.
6. Mustafa M, Rasotgi V, Jain S, Gupta V. Discovery of fifth serotype of dengue virus (DENV-5): a new public health dilemma in dengue control. Med J Armed Forces India. 2015;71(1):67–70.
7. Murrell S, Wu S-C, Butler M. Review of dengue virus and the development of a vaccine. Biotechnol Adv. 2011;29(2):239–47.
8. Rudolph KE, Lessler J, Moloney RM, Kmush B, Cummings DA. Incubation periods of mosquito-borne viral infections: a systematic review. Am J Trop Med Hyg. 2014;90(5):882–91.
9. Jansen CC, Beebe NW. The dengue vector Aedes aegypti: what comes next. Microbes Infect. 2010;12(4):272–9.

10. World Health Organization. Comprehensive guidelines for prevention and control of dengue and dengue haemorrhagic fever, Revised and extended edition. Geneva: World Health Organization; 2011.

11. World Health Organization, Special Programme for Research and Training in Tropical Diseases, World Health Organization. Department of Control of Neglected Tropical Diseases, World Health Organization. Epidemic and Pandemic Alert and Response. Dengue: guidelines for diagnosis, treatment, prevention and control. Geneva: World Health Organization; 2009.

12. De Silva AM, Dittus W, Amerasinghe PH, Amerasinghe FP. Serologic evidence for an epizootic dengue virus infecting toque macaques (Macaca sinica) at Polonnaruwa, Sri Lanka. Am J Trop Med Hyg. 1999;60(2):300–6.

13. Morin CW, Comrie AC, Ernst K. Climate and dengue transmission: evidence and implications. Environ Health Perspect. 2013;121(11–12):1264–72.

14. CDC. Dengue Clinical Case Management (DCCM): Centers for Disease Control and Prevention. 2018 [cited 2019 Mar]. Available from https://www.cdc.gov/dengue/training/cme/ccm/page86100.html

15. Simmons CP, Farrar JJ, van Vinh Chau N, Wills B. Dengue. N Engl J Med. 2012;366(15):1423–32.

16. Hadinegoro SRS. The revised WHO dengue case classification: does the system need to be modified? Paediatr Int Child Health. 2012;32(sup1):33–8.

17. Salgado DM, Eltit JM, Mansfield K, Panqueba C, Castro D, Vega MR, et al. Heart and skeletal muscle are targets of dengue virus infection. Pediatr Infect Dis J. 2010;29(3):238.

18. Srichaikul T, Nimmannitya S. Haematology in dengue and dengue haemorrhagic fever. Best Pract Res Clin Haematol. 2000;13(2):261–76.

19. Seet RC, Quek AM, Lim EC. Symptoms and risk factors of ocular complications following dengue infection. J Clin Virol. 2007;38(2):101–5.

20. Puccioni-Sohler M, Rosadas C, Cabral-Castro MJ. Neurological complications in dengue infection: a review for clinical practice. Arq Neuropsiquiatr. 2013;71(9B):667–71.

21. Ranjit S, Kissoon N. Dengue hemorrhagic fever and shock syndromes. Pediatr Crit Care Med. 2011;12(1):90–100.

22. Kittigul L, Pitakarnjanakul P, Sujirarat D, Siripanichgon K. The differences of clinical manifestations and laboratory findings in children and adults with dengue virus infection. J Clin Virol. 2007;39(2):76–81.

23. Wiwanitkit V. Dengue fever: diagnosis and treatment. Expert Rev Anti-Infect Ther. 2010;8(7):841–5.

24. Malavige G, Fernando S, Fernando D, Seneviratne S. Dengue viral infections. Postgrad Med J. 2004;80(948):588–601.

25. Rajapakse S, Rodrigo C, Rajapakse A. Treatment of dengue fever. Infect Drug Resist. 2012;5:103.

26. Malaysia MoH. Clinical Practice Guidelines. management of dengue infection in adults. 3rd ed. Malaysia: Malaysia Health Technology Assessment Section (MaHTAS); 2015.

27. Tricou V, Minh NN, Farrar J, Tran HT, Simmons CP. Kinetics of viremia and NS1 antigenemia are shaped by immune status and virus serotype in adults with dengue. PLoS Negl Trop Dis. 2011;5(9):e1309.

28. Duyen HT, Ngoc TV, Ha DT, Hang VT, Kieu NT, Young PR, et al. Kinetics of plasma viremia and soluble nonstructural protein 1 concentrations in dengue: differential effects according to serotype and immune status. J Infect Dis. 2011;203(9):1292–300.

29. Blacksell SD, Jarman RG, Bailey MS, Tanganuchitcharnchai A, Jenjaroen K, Gibbons RV, et al. Evaluation of six commercial point-of-care tests for the diagnosis of acute dengue infections: the need for combining NS1 antigen and IgM/IgG antibody detection to achieve acceptable levels of accuracy. Clin Vaccine Immunol. 2011;18(12):2095–101.

30. Peeling RW, Artsob H, Pelegrino JL, Buchy P, Cardosa MJ, Devi S, et al. Evaluation of diagnostic tests: dengue. Nat Rev Microbiol. 2010;8(12supp):S30.

31. World Health Organization. Dengue hemorrhagic fever: diagnosis, treatment, prevention and control. 2nd ed. Geneva: World Health Organization; 1997. ISBN: 92-4-154500-3.

32. CDC. Clinical description for case definitions: centers for disease control and prevention. 2013 [cited 2018 Jun 8]. Available from https://www.cdc.gov/dengue/clinicallab/casedef.html.
33. World Health Organization. Dengue hemorrhagic fever: diagnosis, treatment, prevention and control. 2nd ed. Geneva: World Health Organization, 1997. ISBN: 92-4-154500-3.
34. WHO/SEARO: World Health Organization Regional Office for South-East Asia. Comprehensive guidelines for prevention and control of dengue and dengue hemorrhagic fever (Revised and expanded edition). 2011. ISBN: 978-92-9022-387-0.
35. World Health Organization, Regional Office for South-East Asia, Guidelines for treatment of dengue fever/dengue haemorrhagic fever in small hospitals. New Delhi: WHO-SEARO, 1999.
36. World Health Organization. Dengue Guidelines for Diagnosis, Treatment, Prevention and Control (PDF). Geneva: World Health Organization. 2009. ISBN 92-4-154787-1.
37. Bhatt S, Gething PW, Brady OJ, Messina JP, Farlow AW, Moyes CL, et al. The global distribution and burden of dengue. Nature. 2013;496(7446):504.
38. Mallhi TH, Khan AH, Adnan AS, Sarriff A, Khan YH, Gan SH. Short-term renal outcomes following acute kidney injury among dengue patients: a follow-up analysis from large prospective cohort. PLos One. 2018;13(2):e0192510.
39. Mallhi TH, Khan AH, Adnan AS, Sarriff A, Khan YH, Jummaat F. Incidence, characteristics and risk factors of acute kidney injury among dengue patients: a retrospective analysis. PLoS One. 2015;10(9):e0138465.
40. Shepard DS, Undurraga EA, Halasa YA. Economic and disease burden of dengue in Southeast Asia. PLoS Negl Trop Dis. 2013;7(2):e2055.
41. Stanaway JD, Shepard DS, Undurraga EA, Halasa YA, Coffeng LE, Brady OJ, et al. The global burden of dengue: an analysis from the Global Burden of Disease Study 2013. Lancet Infect Dis. 2016;16(6):712–23.
42. De Paula SO, da Fonseca BAL. Dengue: a review of the laboratory tests a clinician must know to achieve a correct diagnosis. Braz J Infect Dis. 2004;8(6):390–8.
43. Khormi HM, Kumar L. The importance of appropriate temporal and spatial scales for dengue fever control and management. Sci Total Environ. 2012;430:144–9.
44. Soni A, Chugh K, Sachdev A, Gupta D. Management of dengue fever in ICU. Indian J Pediatr. 2001;68(11):1051–5.
45. Nhan NT, Phuong CXT, Kneen R, Wills B, Van My N, Phuong NTQ, et al. Acute management of dengue shock syndrome: a randomized double-blind comparison of 4 intravenous fluid regimens in the first hour. Clin Infect Dis. 2001;32(2):204–13.
46. Wills BA, Dung NM, Loan HT, Tam DT, Thuy TT, Minh LT, et al. Comparison of three fluid solutions for resuscitation in dengue shock syndrome. N Engl J Med. 2005;353(9):877–89.
47. Dmpuk R, Kularatne S. Current management of dengue in adults: a review. Int Med J Malays. 2015;14:1.
48. Ranjit S, Kissoon N, Jayakumar I. Aggressive management of dengue shock syndrome may decrease mortality rate: a suggested protocol. Pediatr Crit Care Med. 2005;6(4):412–9.
49. Thomas L, Kaidomar S, Kerob-Bauchet B, Moravie V, Brouste Y, King JP, et al. Prospective observational study of low thresholds for platelet transfusion in adult dengue patients. Transfusion. 2009;49(7):1400–11.
50. Lye DC, Lee VJ, Sun Y, Leo YS. Lack of efficacy of prophylactic platelet transfusion for severe thrombocytopenia in adults with acute uncomplicated dengue infection. Clin Infect Dis. 2009;48(9):1262–5.
51. Kalayanarooj S. Clinical manifestations and management of dengue/DHF/DSS. Trop Med Health. 2011;39(4 Suppl):S83–S7.
52. Damonte EB, Matulewicz MC, Cerezo AS. Sulfated seaweed polysaccharides as antiviral agents. Curr Med Chem. 2004;11(18):2399–419.
53. Crance JM, Scaramozzino N, Jouan A, Garin D. Interferon, ribavirin, 6-azauridine and glycyrrhizin: antiviral compounds active against pathogenic flaviviruses. Antivir Res. 2003;58(1):73–9.
54. Yin Z, Chen Y-L, Schul W, Wang Q-Y, Gu F, Duraiswamy J, et al. An adenosine nucleoside inhibitor of dengue virus. Proc Natl Acad Sci. 2009;106(48):20435–9.

55. Tricou V, Minh NN, Van TP, Lee SJ, Farrar J, Wills B, et al. A randomized controlled trial of chloroquine for the treatment of dengue in Vietnamese adults. PLoS Negl Trop Dis. 2010;4(8):e785.
56. Miller N. Recent progress in dengue vaccine research and development. Curr Opin Mol Ther. 2010;12(1):31–8.
57. World Health Organization. Dengue vaccine: WHO position paper, July 2016–recommendations. Vaccine. 2017;35(9):1200–1.
58. Monath TP. Dengue and yellow fever—challenges for the development and use of vaccines. N Engl J Med. 2007;357(22):2222–5.
59. Wan S-W, Lin C-F, Wang S, Chen Y-H, Yeh T-M, Liu H-S, et al. Current progress in dengue vaccines. J Biomed Sci. 2013;20(1):37.
60. Van Benthem BH, Khantikul N, Panart K, Kessels PJ, Somboon P, Oskam L. Knowledge and use of prevention measures related to dengue in northern Thailand. Trop Med Int Health. 2002;7(11):993–1000.
61. Abeyasuriya KT, Nugapola NN, Perera MD, Karunaratne WI, Karunaratne SP. Effect of dengue mosquito control insecticide thermal fogging on non-target insects. Int J Trop Insect Sci. 2017;37(1):11–8.
62. Manjarres-Suarez A, Olivero-Verbel J. Chemical control of Aedes aegypti: a historical perspective. Revista Costarricense de Salud Pública. 2013;22(1):68–75.
63. Gulati S, Maheshwari A. Atypical manifestations of dengue. Tropical Med Int Health. 2007;12(9):1087–95.
64. Bhamarapravati N, Tuchinda P, Boonyapaknavik V. Pathology of Thailand haemorrhagic fever: a study of 100 autopsy cases. Ann Trop Med Parasitol. 1967;61(4):500–10.
65. Basílio-de-Oliveira C, Aguiar G, Baldanza M, Barth O, Eyer-Silva W, Paes M. Pathologic study of a fatal case of dengue-3 virus infection in Rio de Janeiro, Brazil. Braz J Infect Dis. 2005;9(4):341–7.
66. Martina BE, Koraka P, Osterhaus AD. Dengue virus pathogenesis: an integrated view. Clin Microbiol Rev. 2009;22(4):564–81.
67. Huerre MR, Lan NT, Marianneau P, Hue NB, Khun H, Hung NT, et al. Liver histopathology and biological correlates in five cases of fatal dengue fever in Vietnamese children. Virchows Arch. 2001;438(2):107–15.
68. Setlik RF, Ouellette D, Morgan J, McAllister KC, Dorsey D, Agan BK, et al. Pulmonary hemorrhage syndrome associated with an autochthonous case of dengue hemorrhagic fever. South Med J. 2004;97(7):688–92.
69. Kuo M-C, Lu P-L, Chang J-M, Lin M-Y, Tsai J-J, Chen Y-H, et al. Impact of renal failure on the outcome of dengue viral infection. Clin J Am Soc Nephrol. 2008;3(5):1350–6.
70. Rao S, Kumar M, Ghosh S, Gadpayle AK. A rare case of dengue encephalitis. BMJ Case Rep. 2013;2013:bcr2012008229.
71. Mallhi TH, Khan AH, Adnan AS, Sarriff A, Khan YH, Jummaat F. Clinico-laboratory spectrum of dengue viral infection and risk factors associated with dengue hemorrhagic fever: a retrospective study. BMC Infect Dis. 2015;15(1):399.

Dengue-Induced Gastrohepatic Complications

2

2.1 Hepatic Complications During Dengue Infection

The liver is one of the common organs involved in dengue infection. Hepatic complications are found in 60–90% of infected patients [1–3]. These atypical complications include hepatomegaly, jaundice, abnormal liver enzymes, and acute severe hepatitis. Most of the dengue cases are presented with mild to moderate elevation of liver enzymes. However, dengue-induced severe hepatitis is associated with ten times rise in transaminases levels and prevails in 3–11% of reported dengue cases [2, 3]. Viral toxicity or dysregulated immunologic injuries are common hepatic manifestations observed in response to DENV.

2.1.1 Clinical Manifestations of Dengue-Induced Liver Disease

Hypochondrium pain, hepatomegaly, and jaundice are three primary clinical manifestations associated with dengue-induced liver disease. As per reported data, the prevalence of jaundice is around 15% in dengue infection [4]. Hepatomegaly is the most common clinical manifestation of hepatic injury which is predominantly associated with DHF rather than DF. Existing data suggest that hepatomegaly can occur in up to 60% patients with DHF as compared to DF where its prevalence is around 40%. A study among Thai population suggests that hepatomegaly is more common among children (90%) compared to adults (60%). Likewise, hepatomegaly is the most recurrent clinical sign observed in DSS, ranging from 30 to 79% of dengue cases [5, 6]. Although hepatomegaly is commonly reported in DHF, it does not affect hepatic enzymes as hepatic enzymes are normal in DHF. This finding was observed among Thai children with DHF, where hepatomegaly was observed in 98% of cases; however, 74% of cases had normal ALT levels [7]. Currently available literature suggests no association between dengue virus serotype and the frequency of hepatomegaly [8]. Encephalopathy with liver dysfunction also accounts up to 8% of dengue cases [9].

© Springer Nature Singapore Pte Ltd. 2021
T. H. Mallhi et al., *Expanded Dengue Syndrome*,
https://doi.org/10.1007/978-981-15-7337-8_2

2.1.2 Impact of Dengue Viral Infection (DVI) on Hepatic Enzymes

A study by Kuo and colleagues suggests that AST levels start to rise from the third day and reach to their peak levels on the seventh to eighth day of illness. However, after reaching to the peak concentration in the blood, ALT levels decline and return to normal over the period of 3 weeks [3]. Severe liver dysfunction that may progress to liver failure is also observed among some patients; this is common during the critical phase of the infection. Similar findings were also observed in another Thai study where dengue infection was the major cause of acute liver failure among children. Other hepatic diseases such as chronic liver disease, hepatitis, and cirrhosis do not prevail in dengue infection [10].

2.1.3 Pathogenesis of Dengue Virus-Induced Liver Disease

Following the mosquito inoculation, infected cells are transported through the lymphatic system to lymph nodes, from where they reach the hepatic macrophages. The DENV replicates in hepatocytes and Kupffer cells. Viral replication in Kupffer cells is limited and occurs in two phases. The phase I is initiated after the onset of infection. The phase I is arbitrated by nitric oxide and INF-α production. On the other hand, phase II is arbitrated by increased levels of IL-6 and TNF-α [11]. The virus attaches itself to the host receptor which is mediated by E protein.

The mechanism of interaction between the DENV and hepatocytes is not clear. However, such interaction of viruses with hepatocyte receptors varies with different serotypes. Studies indicate that the DEN-2 gains entry to HepG2 (human hepatoblastoma cell line) cells via protein 78 (GRP78) [12]. DENV1 uses high-affinity laminin receptors to enter the liver cells [13]. Similarly, heparin sulfate has played an integral role in the entry of dengue serotypes gaining access to HepG2 cells [13].

A cell becomes vulnerable to infection primarily due to the following two factors:

- Ability of virus to enter the host
- Host factors enabling the viral replication

These factors are controlled by virus strains and serotype and the cell type. This can be observed in HepG2 cells that have higher susceptibility to cause infection in the G2 phase of the cell cycle [14]. This is observed among children where they are more susceptible to dengue infections as their cells are in G2 phase of the cell cycle. Other cellular proteins including DC-specific ICAM-3-grabbing non-integrin (DC-SIGN) are also used to gain entry to monocyte-derived dendritic cells [15].

Dengue-induced infection of hepatocytes ultimately leads to apoptosis by several mechanisms. High level of endoplasmic reticulum stress-induced apoptosis is one of the examples to dengue-induced hepatocyte apoptosis [16]. Transcription factor NF-κB activation has also been proposed to induce apoptosis [17]. Similarly, ligand expression induced by apoptosis of tumor necrosis factors is also a related example of apoptosis [18].

CD4 and CD8 cells have an important part in eliminating primary and acute dengue infection. On secondary exposure to dengue virus, the severity of infection is increased as CD4+ and CD8+ cells produce cytokines. During the initial days of infection (day 1–day 3), high serum concentrations of TNFα, IL-2, IL-6, and INF-Υ are observed, whereas the concentrations of IL-5 and IL-10 rise later. Similarly, chemokines having chemotactic activity for T cells, monocytes, natural killer cells, and eosinophils are increased in dengue infection [19].

Major pathological changes include microvesicular steatosis and hepatocellular necrosis, Kupffer cell hyperplasia, Councilman bodies, and cellular infiltrates at portal tract [20]. Hepatocellular necrosis is generally caused in the midzonal areas and centrilobular areas by dengue virus. Autopsy reports from a series of dengue patients in Myanmar showed varying degrees of liver damage, mostly in midzonal and centrilobular areas, with sinusoidal congestion. Clinically significant fibrosis was not reported in this autopsy series [21]. Figure 2.1 illustrates the pathogenesis of dengue-associated liver injury.

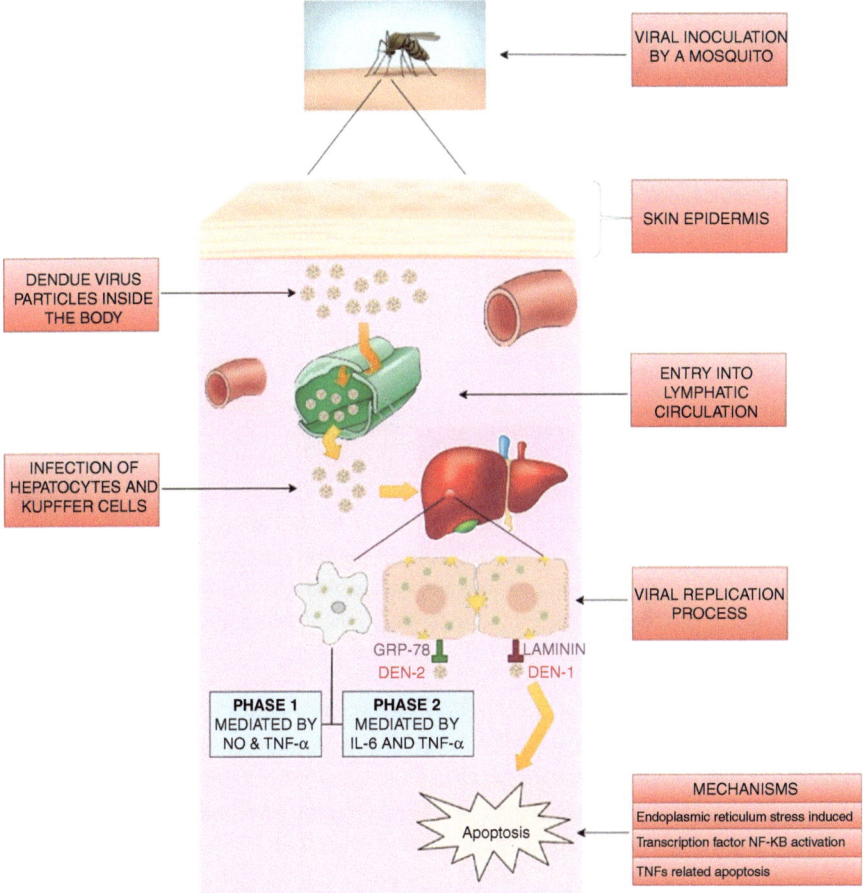

Fig. 2.1 Pathogenesis of dengue virus-induced liver disease

2.1.4   Diagnosis of Dengue-Induced Liver Disease

2.1.4.1 Histological Patterns in Dengue-Induced Liver Disease

Liver biopsy is not possible during dengue infection due to the co-existing coagulation abnormalities, low platelet count, and ascites. Thereby, the major evidence available on dengue-induced liver dysfunction primarily relies on autopsy specimen. Hepatic histological changes include microvesicular changes in hepatocytes, hepatocyte necrosis, hyperplasia, and destruction of Kupffer cells, Councilman bodies, and mononuclear cell infiltrates at portal tract [22, 23]. Midzonal and centrilobular areas are commonly involved in the hepatocyte injury; this is proposed to be due to the sensitivity of liver cells of this area to anoxia or immune response, or perhaps it might be a preferential target zone of DENVs. Autopsy findings of dengue hemorrhagic fever (DHF) show the presence of variable degree of hepatocytes necrosis, mainly in midzonal regions. Previously, it has been reported in literature that replication of dengue viral RNA takes place in necrotic and midzonal hepatocytes [24]. On the other hand, the autopsy report of fatal dengue patients revealed that dengue viral RNA is isolated only from liver tissue and no other organs show viral RNA. Councilman bodies and Torres bodies that are observed in the liver of dengue patients are also reported to be present in fellow fever viral infection.

These findings suggest that the dengue-induced liver pathology is somewhat comparable to liver pathology observed in the early stages of yellow fever. However, dengue-induced liver pathology is less severe and is characterized by extensive hepatocyte necrosis compared to early stages of yellow fever [20]. Moreover, unlike the yellow fever virus where antigen is distributed throughout the cytoplasm, dengue viral antigen is seen as small cytoplasmic foci having large perinuclear inclusions.

2.1.4.2 Biochemical and Laboratory Features of Dengue-Induced Liver Disease

Liver and central nervous system involvement concurrently indicates a poor prognosis in dengue fever. Generally, hepatomegaly and elevated liver enzymes are common features in dengue-induced liver diseases. Hepatomegaly is common in children and is observed with DF and DHF. However, these symptoms are more profound in DF [25]. Moreover other features such as acalculous cholecystitis and impending gall bladder gangrene are rarely observed.

Elevated levels of hepatic enzymes such as aspartate transaminase (AST) and alanine transaminase (ALT) have been reported during the course of dengue viral infection (DVI). A case series of 270 patients have reported that elevated ALT and AST levels were present in approximately 80–90% of subjects, respectively. These elevation in AST and ALT generally ranged from mild to moderately high; however, elevation greater than ten times the upper limit of normal value were found in 11.1% (ALT) and 7.4% (AST) of cases, respectively [3]. Similarly, a study among 169 serologically confirmed dengue cases in Brazil also reported elevated transaminase levels [2]. The study divides participants in four cohorts: cohort A included patients with normal enzyme levels, cohort B patients had increased level of at least one enzyme, cohort C patients had at latest one enzyme greater than three time the upper limit, and cohort D had acute hepatitis with aminotransferase levels greater than tenfold the normal limit. The findings of the study suggest that 3 (1.8%) of study participants belonged to cohort D and 25 (14.8%) belonged to cohort C, whereas 82 (48.5%) belonged to cohort B. Reports suggest that AST abnormalities are more as compared to ALT [26]. This could be explained by release of AST by damaged myocytes which could be the reason of higher levels of AST than ALT during the earlier stage of dengue infection. Moreover, apart from the liver, AST is also released from the heart, striated muscles, and erythrocytes, whereas ALT is primarily released from hepatocytes [27]. Literature suggests that the AST and ALT values are elevated in severe form of dengue compared to uncomplicated dengue [25, 28]. This variation and higher elevation of AST levels compared to ALT in dengue are indicators to distinguish dengue viral infections from other hepatic viral infections.

Other hepatic anomalies during the course of DVI include reduced levels of albumin among patients. Hypoalbuminemia is observed in dengue infection, and its range varies with the severity of disease. An Indian study had reported hypoalbuminemia in approximately 75% of dengue patients [4], while in another study from Hong Kong, the reported prevalence of hypoalbuminemia was 28% among dengue patients [29]. Increase in bleeding tendency has also been reported with elevated liver enzymes [3]. A study has reported that INR values of greater than 1.5 in 11% of patients with dengue might explain increase in bleeding tendencies in such patients [25].

2.1.4.3 Radiographic Findings with Dengue Virus Infection-Induced Liver Injury

Sonographic findings in an acute dengue infection suggest solidification of gallbladder wall. This finding is similar to that present in acute hepatitis, splenomegaly, and ascites [30]. Studies from other Asian countries have reported abnormal liver parenchyma on ultrasound of dengue patients and have attributed these findings to intraparenchymal and subcapsular hemorrhage [31, 32]. A case series of 70 patients reports that 36 patients had hepatomegaly on ultrasonography, whereas clinically evident hepatomegaly was evident among 27 patients [33]. Similarly, around 40 patients had ultrasonographic evidence of ascites, and all these patients had clinically detectable ascites too. Similar findings were also observed by Mia et al. from Bangladesh where ultrasonography findings suggest hepatomegaly, hepatic intraparenchymal fluids, and ascites [34]. The severity of hepatic complications increases with the clinical severity of dengue infection. Hepatomegaly is observed in less than 40% of patients with DHF grade I severity, whereas its incidence increases up to 80% in grade IV severity. Moreover, hepatic intraparenchymal fluid is observed in grade IV compared to 0% in grade I severity, whereas ascites is observed in less than 15% of patients with DHF grade I as compared to 100% of patients with DHF grade IV severity.

2.2   Dengue and Liver Failure

The liver injury in dengue generally varies from asymptomatic hepatic transaminase elevation to fatal acute liver failure (ALF). The incidence of ALF is more common among children as compared to adults [35, 36]. This is evident in a study from Thailand where authors observed ALF among approximately 35% of children aged between 1 year and 25 years, having positive dengue serology [37]. A similar observation was also reported from India where 5 of 27 (18.5%) children had ALF [38]. Tan et al. [39] reported 8 of 155 (5.2%) adult cases had ALF during the course of DVI. The ALF develops around 7.5 day (5–13 day) after the inception of fever. Moreover, ALF may also develop in patients that may be recovering from dengue infection. Dengue has also been reported to cause ALF in patients with underlying liver disease including hepatitis B virus carrier [40].

After an incubation period of 3–7 days, fever develops that lasts for 2–7 days and leads to a critical defervescence phase starting from 3 to 7 days of the illness when plasma leakage is more profound [39]. The severity of the disease is dependent upon the viral load [41]. Dengue has also been associated with worsening of chronic liver disease and acts as a major cause of acute-on-chronic liver failures (ACLF) [42, 43]. It is important to note that the possibility of dengue-induced ACLF should not be disregarded in dengue-endemic areas.

Apart from supportive measures, ALF can be effectively managed with the administration of N-acetyl cysteine (NAC) in adults and children [44, 45]. In a study, NAC was administered to eight adults having varying severities of encephalopathy. Five adults with mild hepatic encephalopathy (grades I–II) recovered completely, while fatality was reported among the remaining three adults with severe encephalopathy (III and IV) [45]. Other agents as molecular adsorbent recirculating system (MARS) have also shown mixed results for the management of ALF [46].

2.2.1   Clinical Relevance of Liver Involvement in Dengue Viral Infection (DVI)

The utility of raised transaminases level for prediction of dengue infection and its severity is not clearly established yet. In a Singaporean study among 690 dengue patients, the levels of AST and ALT could not discriminate between DF and DHF [28]. A study from Lahore, Pakistan, used liver functioning test profile to establish the severity of dengue infection [47]. The study reported that the AST levels were twice higher than ALT levels in dengue patients. However, the levels of AST did not correlate with the development of complication or the duration of hospital stay. On the other hand, the ALT levels had a significant correlation with the development of dengue-induced shock syndrome, septicemia, hepatic failure, encephalopathy, and renal failure. Similarly a Malaysian study have reported significantly higher ALT and alkaline phosphate levels in DHF patients with spontaneous bleeding compared to patients without any bleeding [5].

2.2.2   Management of Dengue-Induced Liver Injury

The management of dengue-induced liver injury revolves around meticulous fluid administration during the leakage phase. As discussed earlier, various studies have reported to use *N*-acetyl cysteine (NAC) in these patients. In a study, five of the eight patients on NAC recovered from hepatic encephalopathy [45]. The use of NAC was rationalized by NAC ability to reinstate hepatocellular glutathione and its potential as free radical scavenger. Moreover, NAC is also reported to improve antioxidant defense. A case series also reported the significance of recombinant factor VII-1 and NAC in non-acetaminophen-induced fulminant liver failure in complicated DHF [48].

Other strategies such as artificial liver support have also been suggested for patients with dengue-induced liver failure. This provides a transitory support to liver function and aids in liver transplantation. One of these temporary liver supports is molecular adsorbent recirculating system (MARS). It has been established that MARS in dengue-infected patients with liver failure helps to rapidly reverse biochemical profile and improves encephalopathy [46]. Single-pass albumin dialysis has also been reported to have beneficial outcomes in dengue-induced liver failure patients [49].

Carica papaya leaf extracts have been extensively used in dengue patients, and studies have reported increase in platelet counts due to this extract. However, its role in hepatic diseases needs further investigations [50]. Celastrol is also used in dengue as it increases INF-α expression along with increased downstreaming of antiviral response. However, its role in liver dysfunction requires further investigation [51]. However, liver transplant is the last option in the case of severe liver dysfunction, but it requires careful consideration due to the complexity of the procedure. Moreover, reports have also suggested that dengue may be transferred through liver transplantation if the donor suffers from dengue [52]; therefore, liver organ transplantation requires careful screening and monitoring.

Dengue vaccination which is currently being employed in different countries has also reported mixed results. Studies suggest that the vaccine (Dengvaxia®) is able to protect from infection in 66% of a subset of 9–16-year-old population. However, the efficacy of vaccine is lower in patients younger than 9 years. Moreover, the vaccine has shown efficacy in patients when given to partially immunized patients post-screening [53].

2.3   Dengue-Induced Gastrointestinal Injury

Dengue infection is notorious for its deceptive nature and affects almost every organ system of the human body [53]. Gastrointestinal (GI) manifestations of dengue were uncommon in the past but are now being increasingly reported due to frequent occurrence of DVI epidemics globally [54]. These GI manifestations include GI bleeding, intestinal perforations, GI ulcers, acute pancreatitis, peritonitis, diarrhea, and rarely acute appendicitis [53–56]. The management of these manifestations presents a dilemma to gastroenterologist [55]. GI bleeding is the commonest form of severe hemorrhage in dengue fever, and there are almost 150,000 known cases worldwide [57]. Intestinal perforations in dengue are very rare and have been reported only in eight patients till date. These perforations include gastric, jejunal, ileal, or appendicular perforations [54, 58, 59].

2.3.1 Pathogenesis of Dengue-Induced Gastrointestinal Injury

Although there is an evidence of intestinal mucosal injury in dengue fever, the exact mechanism of GI manifestations, such as GI bleeding, is not clear [60]. Dengue virus has been suggested to cause intestinal mucosal injury either by direct mucosal invasion or by endotoxin release. Dengue virus also causes intestinal mucosal ischemia as indicated by increased concentration of serum intestinal fatty acid binding proteins, which is a biomarker for intestinal mucosal injury. In severe cases, this intestinal mucosal injury and ischemia may lead to intestinal perforations [54, 60].

2.3.2 Clinical Manifestations of Dengue-Induced Gastrointestinal Injury

The clinical manifestations of GI involvements during the course of DVI include GI bleeding, gastritis, fever with chills, obstipation, ascites, free gas under the diaphragm, bilious vomiting, hematemesis, abdominal pain, abdominal tenderness, thrombocytopenia, decreased hemoglobin levels, increased prothrombin, and partial activated thromboplastin time [57].

2.3.3 Diagnosis of Dengue-Induced Gastrointestinal Injury

Endoscopy is performed to find out GI complications such as GI bleeding, gastritis, and gastric perforations in dengue infection, but there is still no evidence regarding the clinical applications of endoscopic therapy in GI bleeding. The endoscopic findings include hemorrhage, gastritis, gastric ulcer, duodenal ulcer, esophageal ulcer, and upper GI perforations [57].

If the dengue infection has not been diagnosed earlier, then the physician may perform all possible hematological investigations along with malarial parasite, malarial antigen, widal, and dengue NS1 antigen test. On general examination, the patient may appear hypotensive and tachycardic. X-rays of the chest and abdomen and abdominal ultrasonography are performed in conjunction with endoscopy to rule out the other causes of abdominal pain, distension, and tenderness. A plain erect abdomen X-ray may reveal pneumoperitoneum and bilateral free gas under the diaphragm, and ultrasonography may show ascites with internal echoes. In blood investigation, complete blood count may show low hemoglobin levels and decreased platelet count. In emergency, the physician may perform laparotomy for the diagnosis of GI injury and preparation of surgery [54, 61, 62].

2.3.4 Management of Dengue-Induced Gastrointestinal Injury

The function of endoscopic treatment in UGI bleeding remains unknown, but standard endoscopic protocols such as coagulation therapy and mechanical therapy can efficiently treat GI bleeding. However, hemorrhage and GI bleeding may require transfusions of packed red blood cells (PRBCs) and fresh frozen plasma (FFP) [63, 64].

It is recommended to treat peptic ulcers with active bleeding, non-bleeding visible vessels, or persistent oozing endoscopically. Endoscopic injections with agents such as epinephrine (1:10,000 dilution) are effectively used either alone or in conjunction with thermal contact devices to stop or prevent bleeding. The injection therapy creates small needle holes around the bleeding area, but vasoconstriction effect can be used to prevent bleeding. However, the temporary effect of vasoconstriction may not work consistently among patients with bleeding tendencies, such as severe thrombocytopenia and coagulation disorder, and may increase the possibility of recurrent bleeding from the injection sites. This may increase the tendency of blood loss in dengue patients. Few cases of frequent bleeding from the injection sites have been reported in the past [63–65]. Hence, transfusions containing platelet concentrate, PRBCs, and FFP to correct bleeding tendency, anemia, coagulopathy, and hypovolemia are the treatment of choice in dengue patients [63–65].

In severe cases of GI perforations, immediate resuscitation and exploratory laparotomy under platelet cover are to be performed to initiate primary surgical repair of the perforation. The patient should be monitored for 1–2 weeks after surgery, and if the postoperative course is found to be uneventful, the patient should be discharged [54, 55, 57, 60, 62–66].

References

1. Nguyen T, Nguyen T, Tieu N. The impact of dengue haemorrhagic fever on liver function. Res Virol. 1997;148(4):273–7.
2. de Souza LJ, Nogueira RMR, Soares LC, Soares CEC, Ribas BF, Alves FP, et al. The impact of dengue on liver function as evaluated by aminotransferase levels. Braz J Infect Dis. 2007;11(4):407–10.
3. Kuo C-H, Tai D-I, Chang-Chien C-S, Lan C-K, Chiou S-S, Liaw Y-F. Liver biochemical tests and dengue fever. Am J Trop Med Hyg. 1992;47(3):265–70.
4. Itha S, Kashyap R, Krishnani N, Saraswat VA, Choudhuri G, Aggarwal R. Profile of liver involvement in dengue virus infection. Natl Med J India. 2005;18(3):127.
5. Walid S, Sanusi S, Zawawi MM, Ali RA. A comparison of the pattern of liver involvement in dengue hemorrhagic fever with classic dengue fever. Southeast Asian J Trop Med Public Health. 2000;31(2):259–63.

6. Mallhi TH, Khan AH, Adnan AS, Sarriff A, Khan YH, Jummaat F. Clinico-laboratory spectrum of dengue viral infection and risk factors associated with dengue hemorrhagic fever: a retrospective study. BMC Infect Dis. 2015;15(1):399.
7. Nimmannitya S. Clinical spectrum and management of dengue haemorrhagic fever. Southeast Asian J Trop Med Public Health. 1987;18(3):392–7.
8. Limkittikul K, Yingsakmongkon S, Jittmittraphap A, Chuananon S, Kongphrai Y, Kowasupathr S, et al. Clinical differences among PCR-proven dengue serotype infections. Southeast Asian J Trop Med Public Health. 2005;36(6):1432.
9. Wiwanitkit V. Liver dysfunction in dengue infection, an analysis of the previously published Thai cases. J Ayub Med Coll Abbottabad. 2007;19(1):10–2.
10. Poovorawan Y, Hutagalung Y, Chongsrisawat V, Boudville I, Bock HL. Dengue virus infection: a major cause of acute hepatic failure in Thai children. Ann Trop Paediatr. 2006;26(1):17–23.
11. Marianneau P, Steffan A-M, Royer C, Drouet M-T, Jaeck D, Kirn A, et al. Infection of primary cultures of human Kupffer cells by dengue virus: no viral progeny synthesis, but cytokine production is evident. J Virol. 1999;73(6):5201–6.
12. Jindadamrongwech S, Thepparit C, Smith D. Identification of GRP 78 (BiP) as a liver cell expressed receptor element for dengue virus serotype 2. Arch Virol. 2004;149(5):915–27.
13. Thepparit C, Smith DR. Serotype-specific entry of dengue virus into liver cells: identification of the 37-kilodalton/67-kilodalton high-affinity laminin receptor as a dengue virus serotype 1 receptor. J Virol. 2004;78(22):12647–56.
14. Phoolcharoen W, Smith DR. Internalization of the dengue virus is cell cycle modulated in HepG2, but not Vero cells. J Med Virol. 2004;74(3):434–41.
15. Navarro-Sanchez E, Altmeyer R, Amara A, Schwartz O, Fieschi F, Virelizier JL, et al. Dendritic-cell-specific ICAM3-grabbing non-integrin is essential for the productive infection of human dendritic cells by mosquito-cell-derived dengue viruses. EMBO Rep. 2003;4(7):723–8.
16. Su H-L, Liao C-L, Lin Y-L. Japanese encephalitis virus infection initiates endoplasmic reticulum stress and an unfolded protein response. J Virol. 2002;76(9):4162–71.
17. Marianneau P, Cardona A, Edelman L, Deubel V, Desprès P. Dengue virus replication in human hepatoma cells activates NF-kappaB which in turn induces apoptotic cell death. J Virol. 1997;71(4):3244–9.
18. Matsuda T, Almasan A, Tomita M, Tamaki K, Saito M, Tadano M, et al. Dengue virus-induced apoptosis in hepatic cells is partly mediated by Apo2 ligand/tumour necrosis factor-related apoptosis-inducing ligand. J Gen Virol. 2005;86(Pt 4):1055.
19. Lin Y-L, Liu C-C, Chuang J-I, Lei H-Y, Yeh T-M, Lin Y-S, et al. Involvement of oxidative stress, NF-IL-6, and RANTES expression in dengue-2-virus-infected human liver cells. Virology. 2000;276(1):114–26.
20. Rigau-Pérez JG, Clark GG, Gubler DJ, Reiter P, Sanders EJ, Vorndam AV. Dengue and dengue haemorrhagic fever. Lancet. 1998;352(9132):971–7.
21. Aye KS, Charngkaew K, Win N, Wai KZ, Moe K, Punyadee N, et al. Pathologic highlights of dengue hemorrhagic fever in 13 autopsy cases from Myanmar. Hum Pathol. 2014;45(6):1221–33.
22. Bhamarapravati N. Hemostatic defects in dengue hemorrhagic fever. Rev Infect Dis. 1989;11(Supplement_4):S826–S9.
23. Burke T. Dengue haemorrhagic fever: a pathological study. Trans R Soc Trop Med Hyg. 1968;62(5):682–92.
24. Kangwanpong D, Bhamarapravati N, Lucia HL. Diagnosing dengue virus infection in archived autopsy tissues by means of the in situ PCR method: a case report. Clin Diagn Virol. 1995;3(2):165–72.
25. Saha AK, Maitra S, Hazra SC. Spectrum of hepatic dysfunction in 2012 dengue epidemic in Kolkata, West Bengal. Indian J Gastroenterol. 2013;32(6):400–3.
26. Wong M, Shen E. The utility of liver function tests in dengue. Ann Acad Med Singap. 2008;37(1):82–3.
27. Shah D, Rathi P. Dengue-induced hepatic injury. J Assoc Physicians India. 2017;65(12):79–82.

28. Lee LK, Gan VC, Lee VJ, Tan AS, Leo YS, Lye DC. Clinical relevance and discriminatory value of elevated liver aminotransferase levels for dengue severity. PLoS Negl Trop Dis. 2012;6(6):e1676.

29. Chuang VW, Wong T, Leung Y, Ma ES, Law Y, Tsang OT, et al. Review of dengue fever cases in Hong Kong during 1998 to 2005. Hong Kong Med J. 2008;14(3):170.

30. Wu KL, Changchien CS, Kuo CH, Chiu KW, Lu SN, Kuo CM, et al. Early abdominal sonographic findings in patients with dengue fever. J Clin Ultrasound. 2004;32(8):386–8.

31. Pramuljo HS, Harun SR. Ultrasound findings in dengue haemorrhagic fever. Pediatr Radiol. 1991;21(2):100–2.

32. Joshi P, Rathnam V, Sharma S, Balarangaiah G, Kumar G, Bhoi S. USG findings in dengue hemorrhagic fever-our experience in the recent epidemic. Indian J Radiol Imag. 1997;7:189–92.

33. Shukla V, Chandra A. A study of hepatic dysfunction in dengue. J Assoc Physicians India. 2013;61(7):450–1.

34. Mia M, Nurullah A, Hossain A, Haque M. Clinical and sonographic evaluation of dengue fever in Bangladesh: a study of 100 cases. Dinajpur Med Coll J. 2010;3(1):29–34.

35. Giri S, Agarwal MP, Sharma V, Singh A. Acute hepatic failure due to dengue: a case report. Cases J. 2008;1(1):204.

36. Gasperino J, Yunen J, Guh A, Tanaka KE, Kvetan V, Doyle H. Fulminant liver failure secondary to haemorrhagic dengue in an international traveller. Liver Int. 2007;27(8):1148–51.

37. Poovorawan Y, Chongsrisawat V, Shafi F, Boudville I, Liu Y, Hutagalung Y, et al. Acute hepatic failure among hospitalized Thai children. Southeast Asian J Trop Med Public Health. 2013;44(1):50–3.

38. Jagadishkumar K, Jain P, Manjunath VG, Umesh L. Hepatic involvement in dengue fever in children. Iran J Pediatr. 2012;22(2):231.

39. Tan S-S, Bujang MA. The clinical features and outcomes of acute liver failure associated with dengue infection in adults: a case series. Braz J Infect Dis. 2013;17(2):164–9.

40. Agarwal MP, Giri S, Sharma V, Roy U, Gharsangi K. Dengue causing fulminant hepatitis in a hepatitis B virus carrier. Biosci Trends. 2011;5(1):44–5.

41. Thomas L, Verlaeten O, Cabié A, Kaidomar S, Moravie V, Martial J, et al. Influence of the dengue serotype, previous dengue infection, and plasma viral load on clinical presentation and outcome during a dengue-2 and dengue-4 co-epidemic. Am J Trop Med Hyg. 2008;78(6):990–8.

42. Jha AK, Nijhawan S, Rai RR, Nepalia S, Jain P, Suchismita A. Etiology, clinical profile, and inhospital mortality of acute-on-chronic liver failure: a prospective study. Indian J Gastroenterol. 2013;32(2):108–14.

43. Tang Y, Kou Z, Tang X, Zhang F, Yao X, Liu S, et al. Unique impacts of HBV co-infection on clinical and laboratory findings in a recent dengue outbreak in China. Am J Trop Med Hyg. 2008;79(2):154–8.

44. Lim G, Lee JH. N-acetylcysteine in children with dengue-associated liver failure: a case report. J Trop Pediatr. 2012;58(5):409–13.

45. Kumarasena RS, Senanayake SM, Sivaraman K, de Silva AP, Dassanayake AS, Premaratna R, et al. Intravenous N-acetylcysteine in dengue-associated acute liver failure. Hepatol Int. 2010;4(2):533–4.

46. Penafiel A, Devanand A, Tan HK, Eng P. Use of molecular adsorbent recirculating system in acute liver failure attributable to dengue hemorrhagic fever. J Intensive Care Med. 2006;21(6):369–71.

47. Nawaz A, Ahmed A, Alvi A, Chaudhry A, Butt A. Can liver function tests be used as an early marker to assess the severity of dengue fever? A study of prognostic markers of dengue fever: 315. Am J Gastroenterol. 2011;106:S125.

48. Manoj EM, Ranasinghe G, Ragunathan M. Successful use of N-acetyl cysteine and activated recombinant factor VII in fulminant hepatic failure and massive bleeding secondary to dengue hemorrhagic fever. J Emerg Trauma Shock. 2014;7(4):313.

49. Boonsrirat U, Tiranathanagul K, Srisawat N, Susantitaphong P, Komolmit P, Praditpornsilpa K, et al. Effective bilirubin reduction by single-pass albumin dialysis in liver failure. Artif Organs. 2009;33(8):648–53.

50. Kasture PN, Nagabhushan K, Kumar A. A multi-centric, double-blind, placebo-controlled, randomized, prospective study to evaluate the efficacy and safety of Carica papaya leaf extract, as empirical therapy for thrombocytopenia associated with dengue fever. J Assoc Physicians India. 2016;64(6):15–20.

51. Yu J-S, Tseng C-K, Lin C-K, Hsu Y-C, Wu Y-H, Hsieh C-L, et al. Celastrol inhibits dengue virus replication via up-regulating type I interferon and downstream interferon-stimulated responses. Antivir Res. 2017;137:49–57.

52. Gupta RK, Gupta G, Chorasiya VK, Bag P, Shandil R, Bhatia V, et al. Dengue virus transmission from living donor to recipient in liver transplantation: a case report. J Clin Exp Hepatol. 2016;6(1):59–61.

53. Aguiar M, Stollenwerk N, Halstead SB. The impact of the newly licensed dengue vaccine in endemic countries. PLoS Negl Trop Dis. 2016;10(12):e0005179.

54. Kumar P, Gupta A, Pandey A, Kureel SN. Ileal perforation associated with dengue in the paediatric age group: an uncommon presentation. BMJ Case Rep. 2016;2016:bcr2016216257.

55. Ooi E, Ganesananthan S, Anil R, Kwok F, Sinniah M. Gastrointestinal manifestations of dengue infection in adults. Med J Malaysia. 2008;63(5):401–5.

56. Gulati S, Maheshwari A. A typical manifestations of dengue. Tropical Med Int Health. 2007;12(9):1087–95.

57. Zina. Gastroendoscopic manifestations in dengue fever patients. EC Gastroenterol Digest Syst. 2017;1(6):233–9.

58. Mandhane N, Ansari S, Shaikh T, Deolekar S, Mahadik A, Karandikar S. Dengue presenting as gastric perforation: first case reported till date. Int J Res Med Sci. 2015;3(8):2139–40.

59. Jain A, Viswanath S. Multiple jejunal perforations in dengue. Int J Adv Med. 2014;1:153–4.

60. Vejchapipat P, Theamboonlers A, Chongsrisawat V, Poovorawan Y. An evidence of intestinal mucosal injury in dengue infection. Southeast Asian J Trop Med Public Health. 2006;37(1):79–82.

61. Mandhane N, Ansari S, Shaikh T, Deolekar S, Mahadik A, Karandikar S. Dengue presenting as gastric perforation: first case reported till date. Int J Res Med Sci. 2017;3(8):2.

62. Jain AC, et al. Multiple jejunal perforations in dengue. Int J Adv Med. 2017;1(2):2.

63. Chuansumrit A, Chaiyaratana W. Hemostatic derangement in dengue hemorrhagic fever. Thromb Res. 2014;133(1):10–6.

64. Chuansumrit A, Phimolthares V, Tardtong P, Tapaneya-Olarn C, Tapaneya-Olarn W, Kowsathit P, et al. Transfusion requirements in patients with dengue hemorrhagic fever. Southeast Asian J Trop Med Public Health. 2000;31(1):10–4.

65. Chiu YC, Wu KL, Kuo CH, Hu TH, Chou YP, Chuah SK, et al. Endoscopic findings and management of dengue patients with upper gastrointestinal bleeding. Am J Trop Med Hyg. 2005;73(2):441–4.

66. Gulati S, Maheshwari A. Atypical manifestations of dengue. Trop Med Int Health. 2007;12(9):1087–95.

Dengue-Induced Renal Complications

3

3.1 Renal Involvements in Dengue Infection

Renal involvement is one of the most significant target organ involvements in dengue viral infection (DVI). There is a broad spectrum of renal diseases in dengue patients, and such complications include elevation of the serum creatinine (SCr) levels, acute kidney injury (AKI), acute tubular necrosis (ATN), hemolytic uremic syndrome (HUS), proteinuria, glomerulopathy, and nephrotic syndrome [1].

3.1.1 Pathogenesis of Dengue-Induced Renal Diseases

Several mechanisms have been proposed to elaborate the etiology and pathophysiology of dengue-induced renal disorders, including direct action by the virus, hemodynamic instability, rhabdomyolysis, hemolysis, and acute glomerular injury [2]. Since there is no exclusive mechanism that suggests superiority of one mechanism over the other, it is reported that frequently two or more causative mechanisms co-occur at the same time in majority of patients. The available literature show the direct viral invasion of the kidney or the hemodynamic fluctuations during the course of dengue infection as most important attributes of the kidney involvements [3]. In addition to the non-immunological mechanisms, immune system might also play a crucial role in renal intricacies of dengue. Low levels of serum compliment (C3) have been reported in DHF patients especially when shock, sepsis, hemolysis, and rhabdomyolysis are not evident [4]. The hemodynamic instability in dengue patients is believed to be a result of inflammatory cytokines, particularly tumor necrosis factor alpha (TNF-α), interleukin (IL)-6, IL-17, and IL-18, all of which are produced by dengue-infected monocytes and mast cells. These hemodynamic factors lead to renal disorders among patients with dengue infection [5, 6]. Rhabdomyolysis and hemolysis significantly contribute to the development of renal

© Springer Nature Singapore Pte Ltd. 2021
T. H. Mallhi et al., *Expanded Dengue Syndrome*,
https://doi.org/10.1007/978-981-15-7337-8_3

impairments among dengue patients. It has been observed that rhabdomyolysis causes renal dysfunctions through several ways including reduced blood flow to the kidney due to fluid sequestration into damage muscles, direct tubular damage by myoglobin, and intratubular obstruction by myoglobinuria-associated casts in the tubular lumen [7].

Autoimmunity induced by molecular mimicry is another possible mechanism for dengue-associated renal disease since this phenomenon has also been reported in other viral infections, namely, coxsackievirus and Epstein–Barr virus [8]. Autoantibodies against platelets, endothelial cells, and coagulatory molecules have been demonstrated in patients with dengue virus infection and are believed to be a consequence of cross-reactivity to dengue virus antigen, that is, NS1, prM, and E proteins, respectively. These antibodies can cause platelet dysfunction, endothelial injury, and coagulopathy upon binding to their corresponding antigens. Autoimmunity has been reported in dengue patient with serologically and pathologically confirmed anti-glomerular basement membrane (GBM) disease in association with positive p-anti-neutrophil cytoplasmic antibody (p-ANCA) and anti-myeloperoxidase antibody (AMA) on serologic studies. The proliferative pattern with hypocomplementemia has also been reported [9].

3.1.2 Treatment of Dengue-Induced Renal Diseases

The treatment of DVI-associated renal disorders is supportive. Majority of the patients with kidney abnormalities recover with rigorous interventions with fluids and electrolytes. Blood urea nitrogen, creatinine, and creatine kinase monitoring is advisable. Frequent volume status assessment and judicious fluid administration are mandatory. Based on the three randomized controlled trials in children, colloids have no clear advantage over crystalloids regarding the overall outcomes. Therefore, crystalloids are still the fluid of choice in severe dengue infection. Colloids, however, may restore blood pressure rapidly in patients with refractory shock with a pulse pressure less than 10 mmHg [10–12]. Renal replacement therapy (RRT) should be started in patients with persistent volume overload, refractory/severe hyperkalemia, refractory acidosis, or uremia despite a maximally conservative strategy. There is no data regarding dose, modes, or accurate time to initiate RRT in severe AKI patients, which suggests further studies are needed to evaluate the effect of continuous RRT for gradual volume removal on clinical outcomes of such patients. Hemodialysis maybe preferred over peritoneal dialysis due to bleeding disorder accounted by DVI, which may prohibit catheter insertion [13, 14]. The administration of parenteral corticosteroids is debatable in severe dengue cases, and none of the available guidelines recommends their use in such patients [15].

3.2   Dengue-Induced Acute Kidney Injury

Acute kidney injury (AKI) refers to rapid decline in kidney functions characterized by elevated levels of serum creatinine (SCr) and reduced urine output (UO). In recent years, dengue-induced AKI (DAKI) has evolved as an important emerging complication of DVI. The literature reported frequency of DAKI varied widely and the prevalence of DAKI depends on various factors such as disease severity, measures used to account DAKI, time lapse between disease and provision of treatment, and lastly population under assessment [16]. The prevalence of AKI in dengue cases shows great disparity attributed to the methodological variations across literature. Taken together, AKI has been observed in 0.3–14.2% patients with DVI [17, 18]. It has been seen that DAKI can occur at any age, regardless of disease severity. Dengue patients with AKI portend significant morbidly, mortality, and healthcare cost [19]. Recent data also indicate poor prognosis or recovery among DAKI survivors [20].

3.2.1   Pathogenesis of Dengue-induced Acute Kidney Injury

Dengue-induced AKI has diverse etiological factors including direct viral invasion, hemodynamic instability, rhabdomyolysis, glomerulonephritis, hemolytic uremic syndrome, and antigen–antibody complex [14].

3.2.1.1 Direct Viral Invasion and Immune Mechanisms

The direct cytopathogenic influence of the viral attack on the glomerular and tubular cells of renal system is found to be a contributing factor of AKI in DVI. Kidney tissue examination reveals diffused increase in glomerular volume, mesangial and endocapillary hypercellularity, and immunoglobulin M (IgM) deposition in the glomeruli [21]. The viruses have also been detected after inoculation of mouse renal tissue into mosquito cell cultures using an electron microscopy and immunofluorescence technique, thus confirming the presence of viral particles in affected organs. Other mechanism involved in the pathogenesis of DAKI includes immune-mediated physiological responses in the body that occur as a consequence of binding of viral antigens to the glomerular membrane, inflammatory mediators causing tissue injury as a result of cytopathogenic effect of viral antigens, and structural damage caused by immune complexes [22]. Viral antigens have also been detected in renal tubular epithelial cells by immunohistochemical (IHC) and in situ hybridization procedures [23, 24]. However, DENV does not replicate in renal tissues [24]. The association of secondary infection with the development of AKI is well established and is related to the immune mechanisms [18, 25]. Involvement of immune mechanisms in DAKI is explained by antibody-dependent enhancement (ADE). The primary infection with DENV produces subneutralizing antibodies. These antibodies possess high viral attachment efficiency, enhancing internalization of virus into cells through

FCγ receptor (FCγR)-dependent or FCγR-independent mechanisms. The FCγR-dependent mechanism is also proposed to suppress type I interferon-mediated anti-viral responses and promotes the T-helper-2 response, whose antiviral effect is less than the T-helper-1. Eventually, ADE enhances viral replication and cytokine or chemokine production, leading to cytokine-mediated endothelial activation mainly by TNF-α and plasma leakage syndrome [26, 27].

3.2.1.2 Hemodynamic Instabilities

Inflammatory cytokines involving various types of interleukins (IL-6, IL-17, and IL-18) and tumor necrosis factors (TNF-α) are released in dengue as a consequence of severe inflammation. Moreover, the intense inflammatory reaction also activates complement system and platelets that further causes endothelial injury. As a result of forementioned processes, the body becomes hemodynamically unstable, leading to shock and reduced renal perfusion that ultimately causes active tubular injury ultimately leading to AKI [28, 29]. The hemodynamic instability is marked in severe disease (DHF, DSS) and secondary dengue infections, and it might be a possible reason that risks of AKI are higher in such conditions [18, 28].

3.2.1.3 Rhabdomyolysis and Hemolysis

Dengue infection produces muscle injury due to production of myotoxic cytokines, such as TNF and unmediated viral injury [30]. Rhabdomyolysis causes renal vaso-constriction and direct tubular destruction that causes renal damage and ultimately leads to AKI. Muscle injury leads to fluid sequestration into the damaged muscles, followed by intravascular volume depletion. The subsequent reduction in renal blood flow results in activation of a neuroendocrine homeostatic response as well as the release of vasoactive mediators, including endothelin-1, thromboxane A2, and TNF-α, which eventually promotes intra-renal vasoconstriction and AKI. Direct tubular damage can be caused by myoglobin, which is excessively produced and freely filtered through the glomerular filtration slits. Myoglobinuria can also cause intratubular obstruction by forming casts in the tubular lumen [31]. Apart from mus-cle injury, other conditions that cause AKI in dengue patients include acidosis, acid-uria, and hemodynamic instability [14].

3.2.1.4 Autoimmunity

Autoimmunity induced by molecular mimicry is also responsible for dengue-induced renal diseases. This phenomenon has also been reported in other viral infections including coxsackievirus and Epstein–Barr virus [8]. Autoantibodies against platelets, endothelial cells, and coagulatory molecules have been demon-strated in patients with DVI and are believed to result from cross-reactivity to DENV antigen, that is, NS1, prM, and E proteins, respectively. These antibodies can cause platelet dysfunction, endothelial injury, and coagulopathy upon binding to their corresponding antigens. An example of autoimmunity and AKI came from a report of an elderly woman presenting with DHF and AKI in Honduras with sero-logically and pathologically confirmed anti-GBM disease in association with posi-tive p-ANCA and anti-myeloperoxidase antibody on serologic studies [9].

Development of autoantibodies to GBM or neutrophil antigen is believed to be induced by environmental factors including infection [32], which was possibly dengue virus infection in this Honduran patient.

3.2.1.5 Glomerulonephritis and Hemolytic Uremic Syndrome

The development of AKI during the course of DVI is well described in association with the development of glomerulonephritis (GN) and hemolytic uremic syndrome (HUS) [14]. It has been observed that patients who presented with GN caused by DVI developed AKI in later stages [2, 4]. The clinical features of dengue-induced HUS include hemolytic anemia, thrombocytopenia, and AKI [33, 34]. Findings of renal biopsies of patients with HUS along with AKI suggest viral infection due to presence of microtubuloreticular structures and thrombotic microangiopathy [33].

3.2.2   Clinical Manifestations of Dengue-Induced Acute Kidney Injury

Dengue patients with AKI may present without any classical renal signs and symptoms. However, fluid overload is one of the major symptoms of AKI. Due to its asymptomatic nature, AKI in dengue infection is usually neglected if levels of SCr are disregarded [17]. Other symptoms that may associate with AKI include tachycardia, hypotension, rashes, dry skin and mucous membrane, fatigue, and lethargy. It must be noted that dengue infection without AKI also presents with similar symptoms and diagnosis primarily relies on laboratory investigations [35].

3.2.3   Diagnosis of Dengue-Induced Acute Kidney Injury

The diagnosis of AKI is primarily based on SCr and urine output. Existing literature indicate that DAKI has been diagnosed with several classification symptoms [16]. Accurate and timely diagnosis is a pre-requisite to identify AKI cases so that early interventions can be provided to prevent further deterioration of reserve function of the kidney [36]. The diagnosis of AKI conventionally relies on the elevation of serum creatinine with or without decrease in urine productivity. Over the years, the definition of DAKI has evolved from the Risk, Injury, Failure, Loss, End-stage (RIFLE) criteria (2004) to the AKI Network (AKIN) classification (2007) [37, 38]. In 2012, the Kidney Disease Improving Global Outcomes (KDIGO) classification system was established by unification of both previous definitions [39]. Collectively, AKI can be diagnosed as rise in SCr by ≥ 0.3 mg/dl (26.5 μmol/l) in 2 days or elevation of serum creatinine (no less than 1.5-folds from baseline) within 7 days. The different staging of AKI is either based on changes in serum creatinine or change in urine output. The importance of SCr and UO has been confirmed in critically ill patients as both early and lifelong risk of fatality and/or RRT is maximum in patients who meet both criteria for AKI and when these abnormalities persist for longer than 3 days [40]. Since there are several curbs of using SCr and UO as renal function biomarkers, additional biomarkers are required to diagnose AKI especially in conditions where there is a gradual slow change in SCr and UO or where these values give misleading results. There has been substantial development in the discovery and validation of new biomarkers for diagnosis of AKI. The sole purpose of new biomarkers is to substitute or complement serum creatinine to accurately diagnose AKI. The new biomarkers vary in their anatomical origin, biological activity, and time lapse between release of biomarker after initiation of renal injury and ADME (absorption, distribution, metabolism, excretion) profile [41–43]. Apart from timely identification of AKI, most of these new biomarkers also provide evidence about the fundamental etiology and different pathophysiological stages involved in AKI and subsequent renal recovery [44]. The AKI biomarkers can be grouped into different types according to their site of action and function [36] as described in Table 3.1.

The availability of new biomarkers results in early detection of minute alterations in renal profile before elevation of serum creatinine and subsequently identifies patients with indication of kidney injury without evident change in serum creatinine (subclinical AKI) [44]. For accurate definition and characterization of AKI, the 10th Acute Dialysis Quality Initiative (ADQI) Consensus Conference has recommended to utilize traditional biomarkers as well as functional and damage biomarkers [45]. Commercial kits are available for the estimation of various biomarkers such as cystatin C, NGAL, IGFBP7, and TIMP-2. Cystatin C is the only biomarker that is practically being used in some clinical care settings for AKI identification in intensive care units (ICU). Cystatin C is a low molecular weight protein that is naturally produced in all nucleated cells and is also present in tissues as well as body fluids. It inhibits lysosomal proteinases intracellularly and inhibits cysteine proteases extracellularly. Compared to creatinine, cystatin C is considered as a superior marker of kidney function owing to its free filtration from renal glomerulus and lack of tubular reabsorption or secretion. Unlike creatinine, cystatin C is mildly effected by demographic variables such as age, sex, muscle mass, and liver functioning profile. Conversely, cystatin C levels are observed to be different in patients with cancer and thyroid dysfunction, patients taking steroids, and chain smokers [46].

Table 3.1 List of commonly used renal biomarkers

Biomarkers	Effect
Serum cystatin C	Glomerular Filteration Rate (GFR)
Albuminuria, proteinuria	Glomerular integrity
Insulin-like growth factor binding protein 7 (IGFBP-7), tissue inhibitor metalloproteinase 2 (TIMP2)	Tubular stress
Neutrophil gelatinase-associated lipocalin (NGAL), kidney injury molecule-1 (KIM-1), N-acetyl-β-D-glucosaminidase (NAG), liver fatty acid-binding protein (L-FAB)	Tubular damage
Interleukin-18	Intra-renal inflammation

In dengue infection, AKI has been defined by various standards including AKIN, RIFLE, and conventional definition (SCr $\geq$ 2 mg/dl) [16]. The evaluation of renal function and biomarkers has not been included in dengue infection. It might be possible that current estimates of DAKI may change when AKI will be investigated with novel biomarkers during the course of dengue infection. It is suggested that in resource-limited settings, the levels of SCr and UO must be carefully monitored. In addition, differential diagnostic workup should be considered to rule out the other causes of AKI. Urine dipstick testing, urinary microscopy, measurements of urinary electrolytes, renal ultrasound, and biopsies should be considered among patients with severe dengue infection [18, 25]. The particular type of differential diagnostic test would vary from one patient to another and desired clinical outcome. It must be kept in mind that routine baseline tests would always be carried out with more specific and novel investigations.

3.2.4   Management of Dengue-Induced AKI

There is no specific treatment for AKI. The existing literature evaluating DAKI describes conservative management for AKI [18, 20, 25, 47]. Current treatment primarily focuses on the management of underlying cause, treatment of complications, as well as preservance of renal functions. The management of oliguria without volume overload requires provision of fluids, with thorough monitoring to prevent volume overload [48]. Loop diuretics in high doses (furosemide 20–160 mg) are the recommended choice of treatment in AKI. The pharmacokinetic and pharmacodynamic profile of loop diuretics contributes towards their high efficacy, even in severely deteriorated renal function. Although furosemide is most commonly used in all stages of acute kidney injury, its clinical role remains unclear [49–51]. Hyperkalemia with ECG changes, a common side effect of loop diuretics, can be managed with administration of intravenous calcium, sodium bicarbonate, and glucose with insulin. These agents increase movement of K^+ into cells and can be complemented with Kayexalate, which removes K^+ ions from the body. Hemodialysis can be a choice of treatment for severe hyperkalemic AKI [52]. Metabolic acidosis should be corrected with small volume serum bicarbonate with continuous monitoring of fluid volume. Hypocalcemia and hyperphosphatemia can be improved with diet and phosphate-binding agents, such as aluminum hydroxide (500 mg orally with food), for a short period of time, while calcium carbonate (500–1500 mg thrice daily), calcium acetate (667 mg, two/three tablets, before food), sevelamer carbonate (800–1600 mg thrice daily), and lanthanum carbonate (1000 mg with food) can be used for prolong use. All the aforementioned agents used for the correction of hypocalcemia are taken orally. The treatment of hypocalcemia is not initiated in rhabdomyolysis patients unless their symptoms become evident. Since decreased excretion of magnesium by renal tubules results in hypermagnesemia, magnesium-containing antacids and laxatives should be avoided. The dosages of all the drugs that are excreted renally must be adjusted according to the kidney function as estimated by the GFR [35, 37, 50].

Dialysis-dependent DAKI has been described in the literature [53]. Dengue patients with marked elevation of serum creatinine within classification of AKIN-III and RIFLE-F should be considered for dialysis. However, appropriate dialysis modality should be evaluated in future studies. Till date, there are no recommended guidelines for both conservative treatment and hemodialysis of dengue patients, and the consequences of AKI on patient quality of life, survival, and kidney function are unknown.

The evidence of prognosis of DAKI is limited and possesses disparity. Several patients who survived an episode of DAKI showed good prognosis and renal recovery on hospital discharge [47]. However, recent investigations demonstrate that renal recovery following an episode of AKI in dengue patients is unsatisfactory [18, 20]. Persistent renal insufficiency has been reported to prevail in approximately 50% (45–48%) of patients with dengue-associated AKI [20].

3.3 Dengue-Induced Glomerulonephritis

Glomerulonephritis (GN) is a renal syndrome that is defined by inflammation of the glomeruli, filtering network of small blood vessels. Glomerulonephritis is classified on the basis of microscopic appearance of the affected renal tissue. The various types of GN include focal and segmental glomerulosclerosis (FSGS), membranoproliferative glomerulonephritis, membranous glomerulonephritis, IgA nephropathy, minimal change disease (MCD), pauci-immune glomerulonephritis, and crescentic glomerulonephritis. Existing literature has reported various forms of GN during or immediately after the DVI in humans and animal models [1]. Dengue-induced GN appears in both DF and DHF [54, 55].

3.3.1 Pathogenesis of Dengue-Induced Glomerulonephritis

Several possible pathogenic events prevail in viral diseases that are associated with glomerular injury. Such events comprise deposition of antigen–antibody complex in glomeruli, in situ antigen–antibody reactions or cell-mediated injury, viral prompted autoimmune reactions to glomerular structures, host antiviral antibodies, and injury due to various inflammatory mediators produced as a result of glomerular or tubular cytopathic effects [24, 54, 55]. The accumulation of immune complexes in the glomeruli is a well-elaborated mechanism of dengue-induced GN [22]. Immune complex deposits are predominantly composed of IgG, IgM, and C3 and deposit in a coarse granular manner in the mesangial cells of the glomerulus [54]. GN resulting from direct viral entry into renal tissue has been described [1]. Moreover, current studies using immunohistochemistry procedures have reported the presence of viral antigens in kidney tubules of dengue patients [24]. It has also been proposed that DVI is associated with systemic autoimmune disorders, which on rare occasions might involve the kidneys. DVI can also aggravate other immune complex diseases such as systemic lupus erythematosus (SLE) [3].

3.3.2 Clinical Manifestations of Dengue-Induced Glomerulonephritis

Dengue-induced GN presents with hematuria, proteinuria, cast in urine, hypertension, and edema. The incidence of hematuria and proteinuria (both non-nephrotic and nephrotic) in patients with dengue-induced glomerulonephritis helps to differentiate them from typical ATN [56]. Swelling of the whole body and oliguria are two other clinical manifestations associated with dengue-induced GN [55].

3.3.3 Diagnosis of Dengue-Induced Glomerulonephritis

Urinalysis is an important diagnostic aid for GN. The presence of RBCs, proteins, or granular casts in urine is a classical indicator of GN in dengue patients. Ultrasound findings may show normal kidney size but mild ascites may prevail among such patients [55]. Renal biopsy shows IgG, IgM, and C3 deposits along with dense spherical particles in some cases. Low levels of C3 and DENV antigens can be seen in renal tubular epithelial cells of patients with DVI-associated GN [24].

3.3.4 Management of Dengue-Induced Glomerulonephritis

Dengue patients with GN are usually treated conservatively with fluids, antihypertensive medications (furosemide, enalapril), and supportive care [54, 55]. Most of the cases of acute GN are managed with conservative management strategies, but there are some reports where dengue patients with acute GN are treated with hemodialysis [53, 57, 58]. However, the dialysis modality and doses are not yet established for the dengue cases.

3.4 Dengue and Focal Segmental Glomerulosclerosis

Focal segmental glomerulosclerosis (FSGS) is defined by a morphological injury in the renal glomeruli that entails occlusion of glomerular capillary loops by sclerotic material. FSGS is primarily linked with a healing course that directly or indirectly comprises podocyte injury [59]. The collapsing variant of disease is the most destructive form of FSGS and is characterized by at least one glomerulus with segmental or global collapse along with podocyte hypertrophy and hyperplasia [60]. Viruses have been well known to cause secondary FSGS, but there is limited evidence of dengue virus as a causative agent of FSGS. Recent report has identified the association of DENV with collapsing FSGS where virus was positive in renal tissues of six patients. These patients showed bad prognosis, and only one out of six patients had conserved renal function during follow-up [61]. The activation of complement cascade might be a potential link between viral infection and collapsing variant of FSGS that ultimately results in renal tissue deposition. Moreover, the deposition of C3 fraction in the mesangial cells is a specific feature of the collapsing variant of FSGS [62], and it has also been detected in the reported cases [61]. It must be noted that other possible viral etiologies including hepatitis B virus (HBV), hepatitis C virus (HCV), Epstein–Barr virus (EBV), cytomegalovirus (CMV), parvovirus B19 (PVB19), and human immunodeficiency virus (HIV) must be ruled out during the diagnosis of dengue-associated FSGS.

3.5   Dengue and IgA Nephropathy

IgA nephropathy, also known as Berger's disease, is a renal disease that is caused by the deposition of antibody IgA into the glomeruli. IgA nephropathy is the most common cause of primary (idiopathic) glomerulonephritis in the industrialized world. The prevalence of IgA nephropathy in dengue patients is quite rare. However, it has been reported in a patient presented to the hospital with abnormal renal function tests. Patient did not improve renal profile after 2 weeks of hemodialysis and was subjected to biopsy. The diagnosis of IgA nephropathy was based on findings of light microscopic examination which revealed increased mesangial cellularity in glomeruli and mild mesangial matrix expansion. The tubules showed features of ATN and the interstitium showed widespread edema. The direct immunofluorescence examination showed mesangial deposits of IgA (++), IgM (+), and C3 (+), while the evidence of IgG deposits was absent. Serum IgA levels (primarily IgA_1) were also elevated. The patient had received six hemodialysis sessions and two blood transfusions during the 4 weeks of treatment and was discharged from the hospital with normal renal profile and IgA levels. It must be noted that IgA nephropathy caused dialysis-dependent AKI in this case [53]. The underlying mechanism of IgA nephropathy can be understood by the proposition that DVI elicits an altered IgA immune response and results in the formation of nephritogenic circulating immune complexes, which than later deposit in the glomerular mesangium, and the ensuing cytokine and chemokines response results in the mesangial proliferation. This immune-mediated mechanism has been well addressed by the previous investigations [17].

3.6   Dengue and Crescent Glomerulonephritis

Viremia-associated autoantibody formation is rare during the clinical course of DVI. Anti-GBM and ANCA antibodies can be triggered by the DENV. The triggering of these antibodies may lead to AKI associated with crescent glomerulonephritis and is characterized by cellular crescent. A combination therapy consisting of high-dose glucocorticoids, IV cyclophosphamide, and plasmapheresis may reduce the levels of circulating autoantibodies and improve renal function [9].

3.7   Dengue and Systemic Lupus Erythematosus/ Lupus Nephritis

Lupus is a chronic autoimmune disease characterized by overactive and misdirected immune system. The systemic nature of lupus causes involvement of several organ systems including the joints, kidneys, skin, blood, and brain. Systemic lupus erythematosus (SLE) is the most common and severe type of lupus which accounts for 70% of lupus cases [63]. The leading incident case of dengue-induced SLE and lupus nephritis (LN) was observed in 2012. It has been observed that SLE and LN can develop after 1 month of dengue infection [64]. Since dengue and SLE share similar symptomology, accurate diagnosis is of paramount importance. Other causes of SLE including autoimmune diseases must be ruled out before confirming the diagnosis. It must be noted that dengue may trigger SLE in genetically predetermined individuals and increase the immune activity in patients, thus eliciting the disease activity [65]. Dengue viremia may be the trigger for immune complex formation in patients who are predisposed to developing autoimmune disease. However, there is also a possibility that dengue infection triggers dysfunctional immune response, resulting in the development of clinical features of SLE and lupus nephritis in patient with previous subclinical SLE [64]. Lupus nephritis is characterized as classic immune complex mediated renal disease. Around 20% of patients with SLE had positive p-ANCA via indirect immunofluorescence (IIF) [66]. Dengue-induced SLE and LN with p-ANCA positivity has been reported in the literature [66]. Dengue patients with SLE and LN can be treated with infusion of methylprednisolone, oral prednisolone, mycophenolate mofetil, hydroxychloroquine, and antihypertensives, e.g., furosemide. Though it is not clear from existing literature that dengue-induced lupus is de novo or lupus flare, simultaneous occurrence of both disorders cannot be ignored [64, 67].

3.8   Dengue-Induced Nephrotic Syndrome

Nephrotic syndrome is the combination of nephrotic-range proteinuria with a low serum albumin level and edema. Normal urine does not contain protein (albumin), and its presence in urine can be a sign of nephrotic syndrome, indicating the abnormal functioning of kidneys. Proteinuria in dengue has been reported in various small- and large-scale studies with estimated prevalence up to 74% [68]. Mild to moderate proteinuria may present in patients, but proteinuria of 18.3 g/day has also been reported among dengue patients [69]. Proteinuria in dengue is primarily associated with DHF and may use to predict disease severity in dengue [70].

3.8.1   Pathogenesis of Dengue-Induced Nephrotic Syndrome

The primary pathological mechanism of proteinuria in DVI is autoimmune-induced glomerular injury that results in glomerulonephritis. This autoimmune-mediated injury is triggered by viruses. Other postulated mechanisms involve altered filtration of the glycocalyx, as dengue virus and NS1 are known to attach to heparan sulfate, which is part of the glycocalyx [70].

3.8.2 Clinical Manifestations of Dengue-Induced Nephrotic Syndrome

In most of the cases, proteinuria in dengue patients does not appear with evident signs and symptoms. However, nephrotic-range proteinuria may present with frothiness of urine and puffiness of the face. Edema, ascites, and pleural effusion along with high blood pressure may present among patients with very high levels of urinary proteins [69].

3.8.3 Diagnosis of Dengue-Induced Nephrotic Syndrome

Identification and quantification of proteins in urinary sample is the mainstay of nephrotic syndrome diagnosis. Spot urine collection, 24 h urine protein test, urine protein–creatinine ratio (UPCR), and protein dipstick test are some important diagnostic tests that are used among dengue patients for identification of proteins in the urine [70]. Relevant tests to exclude the other systemic causes of nephrotic-range proteinuria must also be performed.

3.8.4 Treatment of Dengue-Induced Nephrotic Syndrome

Existing evidences suggest self-resolving nature of dengue-induced proteinuria without any specific treatment [69]. Persistent proteinuria can be treated with conservative approaches, statins, angiotensin-converting enzyme inhibitors (ACEIs), and corticosteroids [71]. The prognosis of nephrotic syndrome during DVI is favorable. However, extended follow-up must be considered for patients to ascertain the complete recovery.

3.9 Dengue-Induced Hematuria

Dengue-associated hematuria has been frequently reported in the literature with estimated prevalence of up to 31% [68]. The reported prevalence of microscopic hematuria may be 18% in DF and 27% in DHF. It must be noted that hematuria in DVI does not progress to gross condition or AKI [72]. The pathogenesis of dengue-induced hematuria is also attributed to the glomerular injury induced by the immune complexes. Fortunately, in both DF and DHF, microscopic hematuria does not influence patient's renal or general outcome [73].

3.10   Dengue-Induced Electrolyte Disturbances

Electrolyte imbalances are the most common renal symptoms in all types of dengue infection [73]. Of these, hyponatremia is the most prevalent electrolyte anomaly. The levels of sodium are associated with disease severity where lowest levels of sodium have been reported in DSS [73, 74]. It is reported in 14–28% of patients with a serum potassium level of less than 3.0 mEq/L [75]. Mechanism involving hypokalemia is not well-elaborated in the literature. The postulated mechanism of hypokalemia is transient renal tubular destruction that might lead to excessive urinary potassium excretion or the reallocation of potassium within cells [75]. However, several other mechanisms precipitating hypokalemia have also been proposed. Intravenous infusions particularly the lactate-containing solutions have high possibility of precipitating metabolic alkalosis which causes intracellular shift of potassium into the cells. Moreover, metabolic acidosis has also been observed in patients with multi-organ dysfunction [73, 74]. Additionally, increased levels of catecholamines due to stress cause insulin release, or a neutropenia-induced cytokine release has been suggested to increase potassium influx in cells [75]. Dengue-associated hypokalemia can cause neuromuscular weakness. This side effect of hypokalemia is completely reversible with adequate potassium administration without any delay. This infers that hypokalemia and its related effects in dengue patients are due to transient functional impairment and there is no role of renal structural damage in such cases. Another possible reason of hypokalemia in dengue patients might be stimulation of the renin, angiotensin, and aldosterone system (RAAS) as a result of volume depletion. The activation of RAAS in turn increases renal excretion of potassium, thus causing hypokalemia in dengue patients. Conclusively, it might be stated that a variety of different mechanisms contribute to hypokalemia in dengue patients [76].

3.11   Dengue Infection and Chronic Kidney Disease

Dengue infection and chronic kidney disease (CKD) share similar clinical manifestations which makes diagnosis of dengue quite difficult. For example, reduced UO, hemoconcentration, pleural effusions, and ascites are common sign and symptoms in both diseases. In this context, there is high probability of diagnostic delay for dengue infection. Moreover, CKD patients have a narrow window of fluid toleration, and on the other hand, treatment success of dengue patients relies on appropriate fluid resuscitation. Therefore, dengue infection in CKD is a real challenge for the attending physician [77]. Dengue infection in CKD possesses high risk of fluid leakage due to the release of cytokines caused by antibody-dependent enhancement (ADE) during the course of DVI [78].

Dengue in CKD portends considerable morbidity and mortality [79]. Dengue patients with CKD are at profound risk of developing kidney injury and are reported to have high fatality rate [80]. Previous data indicates the use of Ringer lactate, dextran 70, and 6% hydroxyethyl in such patients. However, caution must be exercised with Ringer lactate due to the possibility of hyperkalemia and tissue lactic acidosis in patients with shock. Both these conditions have detrimental effects among patients with preexisting kidney disease [12]. There is a dire need to investigate the suitable type solutions for CKD patients with dengue.

Another challenge during the management of dengue in CKD patients is intrinsic unpredictability of UO measurements. Since treatment success of dengue primarily relies on UO, the prognosis of such patients requires vigilant monitoring. Furthermore, accurate calculations of fluid replacement are obligatory to maintain stable hemodynamics. Hemodialysis, which is the first-line therapy for the management for pulmonary edema and hyperkalemia in patients with CKD, is not an option in DSS patients because of the associated effect on blood profile in terms of thrombocytopenia and altered coagulation profile. Hemodialysis is also practically impossible in DSS patients as it would further compromise the hemodynamic state. Therefore, peritoneal dialysis is the ideal management option in dengue patients with CKD [72].

3.12   Dengue Infection in Kidney Transplant Patients

Kidney transplant patients taking immunosuppressive drugs do not clearly manifest the classical signs of DHF or DSS. It might be attributed to the immunosuppression of dengue-induced cell-mediated (by primary infection) and humoral (by secondary infection) immunity with the use of immunosuppressive drugs [81]. Previous investigations have shown that dengue infection in kidney transplant patients does not progress to DHF or DSS [82, 83]. However, there is a case of DHF following the living donor renal transplant in Singapore [84]. This case is of interest because patients had developed DHF when there was no prior case of dengue transmission in the country. Upon investigation it was reported that 6 months prior to renal transplantation, the patient had suffered from DHF. This raises the possibility whether the allograft could remain infective for 6 months after the resolution of viremia. However, this question lacks support of strong evidence but the propensity of viremia cannot be disregarded for secondary infection. In this scenario, it is advisable to carry out screening of both the donor and the receiver for potential infection. The possible reason of screening might be as any one of them or both might be in the incubation phase of the infection. Such screening must be performed throughout a dengue epidemic or in parts of world where dengue is widespread.

Screening of both donor and recipient is of utmost importance, as DHF may impend danger to both the transplant donor and receiver especially in the postoperative phase. Persistent thrombocytopenia, dysfunctional surviving platelets, and increased fibrinolysis lead to prolonged bleeding, circulatory collapse, and hematoma formation. Hypovolemia in such patients leads to amplified risk of allograft damage. Furthermore, plasma leaking causes hypoalbuminemia that further delays wound healing in the immunosuppressed transplant recipient [84].

There have been increasing reports of mortality and graft rejection among patients with dengue and renal transplant. However, the direct association of dengue infection with these poor outcomes is yet to be elucidated. Azevedo et al. reported five deaths and four graft rejections in relation to chronic allograft nephropathy and infectious causes, but the authors did not related these adverse outcomes with dengue infection. The authors were unable to observe long-term adverse effects on the renal raft or recipient during follow-up. According to their study, it was reported that dengue infections in kidney-transplanted patients follow a benign course. Moreover, there was no abnormal graft function reported during acute dengue infections; however, the slightly increased serum creatinine levels were observed during acute dengue infections. The raised serum creatinine levels were reported to be due to increase plasma leakage. The leakage of plasma results in decreased blood flow towards the kidney [85]. In another study Costa et al. reported ten post-renal transplant dengue patients. Of these, four patients were reported to have DHF without any morality [86]. On the other hand, Prasad et al. reported dengue in eight post-renal transplant receivers, out of which three developed DSS with a fatality of 100% [87]. In another study, the authors reported two severe dengue patients in the immediate post-renal transplant period without any graft rejection and mortality [87]. Since the relationship of dengue infection with poor outcomes among kidney recipients is not well established, it is advised to consider rapid screening tests for DVI before transplantation, particularly during epidemics and in dengue-endemic regions.

3.13 Dengue Infection in Elderly Patients with Age-Related Renal Impairments

Since aging causes changes in the structure and function of the kidney, the propensity of developing hypoperfusion-induced kidney injury is high in this group of patients. Moreover, physiological changes in the elderly may facade some of the clinical indicators of DHF or DSS that causes delayed provision of therapeutic interventions [77]. The existing evidences suggest higher mortality rate and prevalence of AKI in elderly patients with DVI. Vigorous dengue treatment including fluid resuscitation of shock states should be cautiously carried out in such patients [88].

3.14 Dengue Infection-Associated Chronic Kidney Disease

To date, there is limited availability of data that describes the recovery of kidney functions among dengue patients surviving a brief period of AKI [20, 47]. In our previous investigation, a high prevalence of dengue-induced AKI and its relationship with a subsequent risk of renal deterioration were observed. Depending on the criteria used, the extent of renal recovery differs among AKI survivors with majority of patients achieving less than 25% of baseline SCr. A significant number of patients had eGFR compatible with the criteria of CKD. However, this study lacks appropriate diagnosis of CKD, and association of dengue infection with CKD cannot be strengthened merely on eGFR estimation. This study found various features such as renal insufficiencies during hospital discharge, multiple organ dysfunctions, old age, female gender, and diabetes mellitus in association with short-term adverse renal outcomes [20]. This data suggest that dengue patients with AKI deserve a careful and long-term medical follow-up, especially under nephrology care. In this context, there is a dire need for appropriately powered multicenter trials with longer follow-up period to validate these findings and to clarify the utility of criteria for renal recovery in dengue patients.

References

1. Lizarraga KJ, Nayer A. Dengue-associated kidney disease. J Nephropathol. 2014;3(2):57.
2. Lima EQ, Nogueira ML, editors. Viral hemorrhagic fever–induced acute kidney injury. Semin Nephrol. 2008;28(4):409–15.
3. Wiwanitkit V. Dengue nephropathy: immunopathology and immune complex involvement. Saudi J Kidney Dis Transpl. 2016;27(6):1280.
4. Bhagat M, Zaki SA, Sharma S, Manglani MV. Acute glomerulonephritis in dengue haemorrhagic fever in the absence of shock, sepsis, haemolysis or rhabdomyolysis. Paediatr Int Child Health. 2012;32(3):161–3.
5. Pagliari C, Quaresma JAS, Kanashiro-Galo L, de Carvalho LV, Vitoria WO, da Silva WLF, et al. Human kidney damage in fatal dengue hemorrhagic fever results of glomeruli injury mainly induced by IL17. J Clin Virol. 2016;75:16–20.
6. Brown MG, Hermann LL, Issekutz AC, Marshall JS, Rowter D, Al-Afif A, et al. Dengue virus infection of mast cells triggers endothelial cell activation. J Virol. 2011;85(2):1145–50.
7. Puapatanakul P, Lumlertgul N, Srisawat N. Renal dysfunction in dengue virus infection. Southeast Asian J Trop Med Public Health. 2017;48:160–70.
8. Lin Y-S, Yeh T-M, Lin C-F, Wan S-W, Chuang Y-C, Hsu T-K, et al. Molecular mimicry between virus and host and its implications for dengue disease pathogenesis. Exp Biol Med. 2011;236(5):515–23.
9. Lizarraga KJ, Florindez JA, Daftarian P, Andrews DM, Ortega LM, Mendoza JM, et al. Anti-GBM disease and ANCA during dengue infection. Clin Nephrol. 2015;83(2):104–10.
10. Dung N, Day N, Tam D, Loan H, Chau H, Minh L, et al. Fluid replacement in dengue shock syndrome: a randomized, double-blind comparison of four intravenous-fluid regimens. Clin Infect Dis. 1999;29(4):787–94.
11. Nhan NT, Phuong CXT, Kneen R, Wills B, Van My N, Phuong NTQ, et al. Acute management of dengue shock syndrome: a randomized double-blind comparison of 4 intravenous fluid regimens in the first hour. Clin Infect Dis. 2001;32(2):204–13.
12. Wills BA, Dung NM, Loan HT, Tam DT, Thuy TT, Minh LT, et al. Comparison of three fluid solutions for resuscitation in dengue shock syndrome. N Engl J Med. 2005;353(9):877–89.
13. John S, Eckardt K-U. Renal replacement strategies in the ICU. Chest. 2007;132(4):1379–88.
14. Oliveira JFP, Burdmann EA. Dengue-associated acute kidney injury. Clin Kidney J. 2015;8(6):681–5.
15. Zhang F, Kramer CV. Corticosteroids for dengue infection. Cochrane Database Syst Rev. 2014;2014(7):CD003488.
16. Mallhi TH, Khan AH, Sarriff A, Adnan AS, Khan YH, Jummaat F. Defining acute kidney injury in dengue viral infection by conventional and novel classification systems (AKIN and RIFLE): a comparative analysis. Postgrad Med J. 2016;92(1084):78–86.

17. Mallhi TH, Sarriff A, Adnan AS, Khan YH, Hamzah AA, Jummaat F, et al. Dengue-induced Acute Kidney Injury (DAKI): a neglected and fatal complication of dengue viral infection—a systematic review. J Coll Physicians Surg Pak. 2015;25(11):828–34.
18. Mallhi TH, Khan AH, Adnan AS, Sarriff A, Khan YH, Jummaat F. Incidence, characteristics and risk factors of acute kidney injury among dengue patients: a retrospective analysis. PLoS One. 2015;10(9):e0138465.
19. Mallhi TH, Khan AH, Sarriff A, Adnan AS, Khan YH. Determinants of mortality and prolonged hospital stay among dengue patients attending tertiary care hospital: a cross-sectional retrospective analysis. BMJ Open. 2017;7(7):e016805.
20. Mallhi TH, Khan AH, Adnan AS, Sarriff A, Khan YH, Gan SH. Short-term renal outcomes following acute kidney injury among dengue patients: a follow-up analysis from large prospective cohort. PLoS One. 2018;13(2):e0192510.
21. Barreto D, Takiya C, Paes MV, Farias-Filho J, Pinhao AT, Alves A, et al. Histopathological aspects of Dengue-2 virus infected mice tissues and complementary virus isolation. J Submicrosc Cytol Pathol. 2004;36:121–30.
22. Glassock R. Immune complex-induced glomerular injury in viral diseases: an overview. Kidney Int Suppl. 1991;35:S5.
23. Basílio-de-Oliveira C, Aguiar G, Baldanza M, Barth O, Eyer-Silva W, Paes M. Pathologic study of a fatal case of dengue-3 virus infection in Rio de Janeiro, Brazil. Braz J Infect Dis. 2005;9(4):341–7.
24. Jessie K, Fong MY, Devi S, Lam SK, Wong KT. Localization of dengue virus in naturally infected human tissues, by immunohistochemistry and in situ hybridization. J Infect Dis. 2004;189(8):1411–8.
25. Diptyanusa A, Phumratanaprapin W, Phonrat B, Poovorawan K, Hanboonkunupakarn B, Sriboonvorakul N. Characteristics and associated factors of acute kidney injury among adult dengue patients: a retrospective single-center study. PLoS One. 2019;14(1):e0210360.
26. Wan S-W, Lin C-F, Yeh T-M, Liu C-C, Liu H-S, Wang S, et al. Autoimmunity in dengue pathogenesis. J Formos Med Assoc. 2013;112(1):3–11.
27. Green S, Rothman A. Immunopathological mechanisms in dengue and dengue hemorrhagic fever. Curr Opin Infect Dis. 2006;19(5):429–36.
28. Pang T, Cardosa MJ, Guzman MG. Of cascades and perfect storms: the immunopathogenesis of dengue haemorrhagic fever-dengue shock syndrome (DHF/DSS). Immunol Cell Biol. 2007;85(1):43–5.
29. Nascimento EJ, Hottz ED, Garcia-Bates TM, Bozza F, Marques ET Jr, Barratt-Boyes SM. Emerging concepts in dengue pathogenesis: interplay between plasmablasts, platelets, and complement in triggering vasculopathy. Crit Rev Immunol. 2014;34(3):227–40.
30. Gandini M, Reis SRNI, Torrentes-Carvalho A, Azeredo EL, Marcos da Silva S, Galler R, et al. Dengue-2 and yellow fever 17DD viruses infect human dendritic cells, resulting in an induction of activation markers, cytokines and chemokines and secretion of different TNF-α and IFN-α profiles. Mem Inst Oswaldo Cruz. 2011;106(5):594–605.
31. Bosch X, Poch E, Grau JM. Rhabdomyolysis and acute kidney injury. N Engl J Med. 2009;361(1):62–72.
32. Tarzi RM, Cook HT, Pusey CD. Crescentic glomerulonephritis: new aspects of pathogenesis. Semin Nephrol. 2011;31(4):361–8.
33. Wiersinga WJ, Scheepstra CG, Kasanardjo JS, de Vries PJ, Zaaijer H, Geerlings SE. Dengue fever–induced hemolytic uremic syndrome. Clin Infect Dis. 2006;43(6):800–1.
34. Aroor S, Kumar S, Mundkur S, Kumar M. Hemolytic uremic syndrome associated with dengue fever in an adolescent girl. Indian J Pediatr. 2014;81(12):1397–8.
35. Schrier RW, Wang W, Poole B, Mitra A. Acute renal failure: definitions, diagnosis, pathogenesis, and therapy. J Clin Invest. 2004;114(1):5–14.
36. Ostermann M, Joannidis M. Acute kidney injury 2016: diagnosis and diagnostic workup. Crit Care. 2016;20(1):299.
37. Bellomo R, Ronco C, Kellum JA, Mehta RL, Palevsky P. Acute renal failure–definition, outcome measures, animal models, fluid therapy and information technology needs: the Second

International Consensus Conference of the Acute Dialysis Quality Initiative (ADQI) Group. Crit Care. 2004;8(4):R204.

38. Mehta RL, Kellum JA, Shah SV, Molitoris BA, Ronco C, Warnock DG, et al. Acute kidney injury network: report of an initiative to improve outcomes in acute kidney injury. Crit Care. 2007;11(2):R31.

39. Kellum JA, Lameire N, Aspelin P, Barsoum RS, Burdmann EA, Goldstein SL, et al. Kidney disease: improving global outcomes (KDIGO) acute kidney injury work group. KDIGO clinical practice guideline for acute kidney injury. Kidney Int Suppl. 2012;2(1):1–138.

40. Kellum JA, Sileanu FE, Murugan R, Lucko N, Shaw AD, Clermont G. Classifying AKI by urine output versus serum creatinine level. J Am Soc Nephrol. 2015;26(9):2231–8.

41. Prowle JR, Liu Y-L, Licari E, Bagshaw SM, Egi M, Haase M, et al. Oliguria as predictive biomarker of acute kidney injury in critically ill patients. Crit Care. 2011;15(4):R172.

42. Hawkins R. New biomarkers of acute kidney injury and the cardio-renal syndrome. Korean J Lab Med. 2011;31(2):72–80.

43. Ricci Z, Cruz DN, Ronco C. Classification and staging of acute kidney injury: beyond the RIFLE and AKIN criteria. Nat Rev Nephrol. 2011;7(4):201.

44. Vanmassenhove J, Vanholder R, Nagler E, Van Biesen W. Urinary and serum biomarkers for the diagnosis of acute kidney injury: an in-depth review of the literature. Nephrol Dial Transplant. 2012;28(2):254–73.

45. Murray PT, Mehta RL, Shaw A, Ronco C, Endre Z, Kellum JA, et al. Potential use of biomarkers in acute kidney injury: report and summary of recommendations from the 10th Acute Dialysis Quality Initiative consensus conference. Kidney Int. 2014;85(3):513–21.

46. Zhang Z, Lu B, Sheng X, Jin N. Cystatin C in prediction of acute kidney injury: a systemic review and meta-analysis. Am J Kidney Dis. 2011;58(3):356–65.

47. Khalil MA, Sarwar S, Chaudry MA, Maqbool B, Khalil Z, Tan J, et al. Acute kidney injury in dengue virus infection. Nephrol Dial Transplant Plus. 2012;5(5):390–4.

48. Prowle JR, Echeverri JE, Ligabo EV, Ronco C, Bellomo R. Fluid balance and acute kidney injury. Nat Rev Nephrol. 2010;6(2):107.

49. Lameire NH, Bagga A, Cruz D, De Maeseneer J, Endre Z, Kellum JA, et al. Acute kidney injury: an increasing global concern. Lancet. 2013;382(9887):170–9.

50. Bellomo R, Kellum JA, Ronco C. Acute kidney injury. Lancet. 2012;380(9843):756–66.

51. Ho K, Power B. Benefits and risks of furosemide in acute kidney injury. Anaesthesia. 2010;65(3):283–93.

52. Evans KJ, Greenberg A. Hyperkalemia: a review. J Intensive Care Med. 2005;20(5):272–90.

53. Upadhaya BK, Sharma A, Khaira A, Dinda AK, Agarwal SK, Tiwari SC. Transient IgA nephropathy with acute kidney injury in a patient with dengue fever. Saudi J Kidney Dis Transplant. 2010;21(3):521.

54. Ghosh M, Banerjee M, Das S, Chakraborty S. Dengue infection with multi-organ involvement. Scand J Infect Dis. 2011;43(4):316–8.

55. Meena K, Kumar P, Paul P. Acute glomerulonephritis in dengue hemorrhagic fever: a rare case report. Ann Trop Med Public Health. 2013;6(5):581.

56. Kupin WL. Viral-associated GN: hepatitis B and other viral infections. Clin J Am Soc Nephrol. 2017;12(9):1529–33.

57. Nair VR, Unnikrishnan D, Satish B, Sahadulla M. Acute renal failure in dengue fever in the absence of bleeding manifestations or shock. Infect Dis Clin Pract. 2005;13(3):142–3.

58. Lima EQ, Gorayeb FS, Zanon JR, Nogueira ML, Ramalho HJ, Burdmann EA. Dengue haemorrhagic fever-induced acute kidney injury without hypotension, haemolysis or rhabdomyolysis. Nephrol Dial Transplant. 2007;22(11):3322–6.

59. Angioi A, Pani A. FSGS: from pathogenesis to the histological lesion. J Nephrol. 2016;29(4):517–23.

60. D'Agati VD, Fogo AB, Bruijn JA, Jennette JC. Pathologic classification of focal segmental glomerulosclerosis: a working proposal. Am J Kidney Dis. 2004;43(2):368–82.

61. Stanley de Almeida A, Cordeiro TM, Belisário AR, de Almeida Araújo RF, Marinho PES, Kroon EG, et al. First report of collapsing variant of focal segmental glomerulosclerosis triggered by arbovirus: dengue and Zika virus infection. Clin Kidney J. 2018;11(3):1.
62. Lum L, Ng C, Khoo E. Managing dengue fever in primary care: a practical approach. Malays Fam Physician. 2014;9(2):2.
63. Maidhof W, Hilas O. Lupus: an overview of the disease and management options. Pharm Ther. 2012;37(4):240.
64. Rajadhyaksha A, Mehra S. Dengue fever evolving into systemic lupus erythematosus and lupus nephritis: a case report. Lupus. 2012;21(9):999–1002.
65. de Souza SP, de Moura CGG. Dengue mimicking a lupus flare. J Clin Rheumatol. 2010;16(1):47–8.
66. Sen D, Isenberg DA. Antineutrophil cytoplasmic autoantibodies in systemic lupus erythematosus. Lupus. 2003;12(9):651–8.
67. Talib S, Bhattu S, Bhattu R, Deshpande S, Dahiphale D. Dengue fever triggering systemic lupus erythematosus and lupus nephritis: a case report. Int Med Case Rep J. 2013;6:71.
68. Horvath R, McBride WJ, Hanna JN. Clinical features of hospitalized patients during dengue-3 epidemic in far North Queensland. Dengue Bulletin. 1999;23:24–29.
69. Ikhtaire S. Nephrotic-range proteinuria in a patient with dengue fever: a case report from Bangladesh. IMC J Med Sci. 2018;12(2):86–9.
70. Vasanwala FF, Thein T-L, Leo Y-S, Gan VC, Hao Y, Lee LK, et al. Predictive value of proteinuria in adult dengue severity. PLoS Negl Trop Dis. 2014;8(2):e2712.
71. Hull RP, Goldsmith DJ. Nephrotic syndrome in adults. BMJ. 2008;336(7654):1185–9.
72. Gurugama P, Jayarajah U, Wanigasuriya K, Wijewickrama A, Perera J, Seneviratne SL. Renal manifestations of dengue virus infections. J Clin Virol. 2018;101:1–6.
73. Lumpaopong A, Kaewplang P, Watanaveeradej V, Thirakhupt P, Chamnanvanakij S, Srisuwan K, et al. Electrolyte disturbances and abnormal urine analysis in children with dengue infection. Southeast Asian J Trop Med Public Health. 2010;41(1):72.
74. Ying R, Tang X, Zhang F, Cai W, Chen Y, Wang J, et al. Clinical characteristics of the patients with dengue fever seen from 2002 to 2006 in Guangzhou. Zhonghua shi yan he lin chuang bing du xue za zhi = Zhonghua shiyan he linchuang bingduxue zazhi = Chin J Exp Clin Virol. 2007;21(2):123–5.
75. Jha S, Ansari M. Dengue infection causing acute hypokalemic quadriparesis. Neurol India. 2010;58(4):592.
76. Hira HS, Kaur A, Shukla A. Acute neuromuscular weakness associated with dengue infection. J Neurosci Rural Pract. 2012;3(1):36.
77. Kuo M-C, Chang J-M, Lu P-L, Chiu Y-W, Chen H-C, Hwang S-J. Difficulty in diagnosis and treatment of dengue hemorrhagic fever in patients with chronic renal failure: report of three cases of mortality. Am J Trop Med Hyg. 2007;76(4):752–6.
78. Pecoits-Filho R, Heimbürger O, Bárány P, Suliman M, Fehrman-Ekholm I, Lindholm B, et al. Associations between circulating inflammatory markers and residual renal function in CRF patients. Am J Kidney Dis. 2003;41(6):1212–8.
79. Kuo M-C, Lu P-L, Chang J-M, Lin M-Y, Tsai J-J, Chen Y-H, et al. Impact of renal failure on the outcome of dengue viral infection. Clin J Am Soc Nephrol. 2008;3(5):1350–6.
80. Lee K, Liu J-W, Yang KD. Clinical characteristics, risk factors, and outcomes in adults experiencing dengue hemorrhagic fever complicated with acute renal failure. Am J Trop Med Hyg. 2009;80(4):651–5.
81. Halstead SB. Pathogenesis of dengue: challenges to molecular biology. Science. 1988;239(4839):476–81.
82. Renaud CJ, Manjit K, Pary S. Dengue has a benign presentation in renal transplant patients: a case series. Nephrology. 2007;12(3):305–7.
83. Chacko B, John GT, Jacob CK, Vijayakumar T. Dengue shock syndrome in a renal transplant recipient. Transplantation. 2004;77(4):634–5.

84. Tan FL-S, Loh DL, Prabhakaran K. Dengue haemorrhagic fever after living donor renal transplantation. Nephrol Dial Transplant. 2005;20(2):447–8.
85. Azevedo LS, Carvalho DB, Matuck T, Alvarenga MF, Morgado L, Magalhaes I, et al. Dengue in renal transplant patients: a retrospective analysis. Transplantation. 2007;84(6):792–4.
86. Costa SD, da Silva GB Jr, Jacinto CN, Martiniano LVM, Amaral YS, Paes FJVN, et al. Dengue fever among renal transplant recipients: a series of 10 cases in a tropical country. Am J Trop Med Hyg. 2015;93(2):394–6.
87. Prasad N, Bhadauria D, Sharma R, Gupta A, Kaul A, Srivastava A. Dengue virus infection in renal allograft recipients: a case series during 2010 outbreak. Transpl Infect Dis. 2012;14(2):163–8.
88. Lee K, Liu J-W, Yang KD. Clinical and laboratory characteristics and risk factors for fatality in elderly patients with dengue hemorrhagic fever. Am J Trop Med Hyg. 2008;79(2):149–53.

Dengue-Induced Cardiac Complications 4

4.1 Cardiac Involvements in Dengue Infection

Dengue-induced cardiac injury is an uncommon intricacy of dengue viral infection (DVI) and has been previously reported in the healthcare centers receiving a large number of dengue patients. Cardiac involvement is thought to occur more in the severe forms of disease such as DHF and DSS. Clinical features of cardiac involvement vary widely: from transient and self-limiting to severe and fatal myocarditis. Arrhythmias, hypotension, pericarditis, rhythm abnormalities, myocarditis, and myocardial depression-producing symptoms of shock and heart failure have been reported previously [1, 2]. Cardiac dysfunction may also play a role in pathogenesis of shock. The diagnosis of cardiac injury during the dengue infection is of utmost importance to avoid hemodynamic collapse [3].

The association of dengue virus (DENV) serotypes with various complications should be while managing the dengue patients. Existing data indicate the association of DENV2 and DENV3 with atypical complications of DVI. Both these viruses have been found to be associated with asymptomatic myocarditis and myocardial dysfunction among patients with DSS and DHF [3, 4]. There are no reports yet on cardiac involvement in DENV1 or DENV4 infection, and there is not enough evidence to determine whether only one or two particular serotypes are associated with cardiac injury [4]. Though association of severe dengue with secondary infection is well established [5], whether cardiac involvement is more common in secondary infection is still unknown. The variation in cardiac involvement among epidemics [6] is thought to be a result of difference in antigenicity related to serotypes.

4.2 Pathogenesis

The exact mechanisms leading to cardiac involvement in dengue infection are not clearly understood. However, two mechanisms of cardiac injury are proposed: (1) the first includes direct invasion and damage to cardiac myocytes by DENV and (2)

© Springer Nature Singapore Pte Ltd. 2021
T. H. Mallhi et al., *Expanded Dengue Syndrome*,
https://doi.org/10.1007/978-981-15-7337-8_4

the second includes cytokine-induced myocardial cell injury caused by an ongoing inflammation [7, 8].

Various inflammatory mediators, such as cytokines, tumor necrosis factor-α, interleukins (IL-1, IL-2, IL-6, IL-13, IL-18, etc.), and cytotoxic factors (such as free radicals), lead to increased capillary permeability and may play a vital role in the pathogenesis of acute myocarditis [9–14]. It is also suggested that derangements of calcium ion storage in the myocytes directly contribute to the causation of myocarditis [15, 16]. Some major pathological mechanisms of cardiac injury in DENV infection are shown in Fig. 4.1.

Upon entry into the body, DENV is taken up by the macrophages which ultimately cause the activation of T cells. These activated T cells release a large number of inflammatory mediators and cause the activation of complement system pathways (C3a and C5a) [17]. This leads to inflammation and necrosis of the endothelial cell lining of blood vessels causing increased capillary permeability and vascular leakage. The plasma leakage in the interstitial spaces of myocytes causes myocardial interstitial edema leading to the impaired myocardial contraction and decreased overall function [17]. The plasma leakage also causes decreased intravascular blood volume leading to impaired coronary circulation. Certain inflammatory mediators released also cause alteration in electrical conduction of heart and suppression of cardiac contractility which leads to conduction block and arrhythmias.

The release of inflammatory mediators is often a sign of severe form of disease and associated with high incidence of cardiac involvement in patients with severe dengue infection. Cardiac injury, often transient, can sometimes be severe and can cause progressive and unmanageable acute heart failure, global hypokinesia, and cardiac dilatation [3, 18, 19]. Impaired circulation also causes lactic acidosis which can contribute to myocardial depression in severe cases [20].

PATHOLOGICAL MECHANISMS OF CARDIAC INVOLVEMENT IN DENV INFECTION

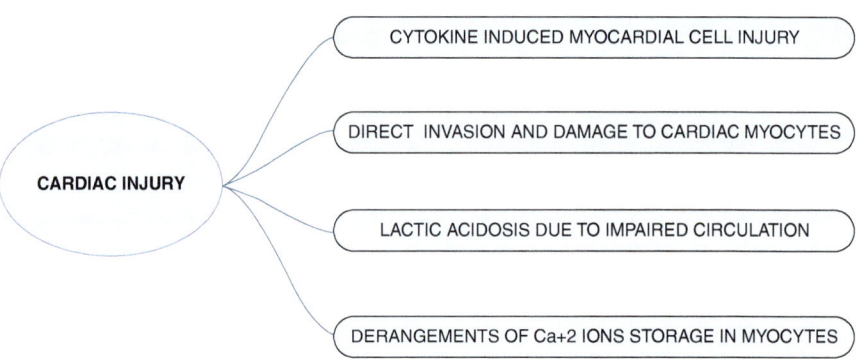

Fig. 4.1 Pathological mechanisms of cardiac involvement during dengue infection

4.3 Clinical Manifestations

Cardiac manifestations in dengue infection are diverse and can range from asymptomatic bradycardia to life-threatening myocarditis and myocardial edema. Most of the clinical symptoms are self-limiting and resolve with the passage of time. Most common symptoms of cardiac involvement in dengue infection include chest pain, palpitations, pleurisy, irregularities of pulse, sinus bradycardia, sinus tachycardia, tachyarrhythmias (such as atrial fibrillation), pericardial effusion, wall hypokinesia, hypotension, pulmonary edema, elevation of cardiac enzymes, and features of shock [21, 22].

The occurrence of these clinical symptoms has been associated with the severity of disease. There is growing body of evidences suggesting the relationship between disease severity and occurrence of cardiac symptoms. Patients with severe forms of DVI (DHF and DSS) possess higher risks of developing cardiac manifestations as compared to those with DF. Severe cases of dengue infection are associated with fluid accumulation resulting in respiratory distress which is further correlated with cardiac manifestations [23].

4.3.1 Electrocardiogram (ECG) Abnormalities

ECG abnormalities among patients suffering from DVI are also used to indicate cardiac involvement [24]. A wide range of ECG abnormalities have been reported in dengue infection, such as rate and rhythm, heart block, wave form, and voltage abnormalities [21, 22, 25–35]. ECG abnormalities like those in myocardial infarction have also been reported [34]. Some of the rhythm abnormalities identified in dengue patients include bradycardia [25], sinoatrial block [26], impaired atrioventricular conduction [21, 26], second-degree heart block [27, 28], complete heart block [28], monomorphic premature ventricular contractions [27], atrial flutter [29], transient and persistent atrial fibrillation [30, 31], self-limiting arrhythmias [22], and uniform ventricular ectopics progressing to ventricular bigeminy [32].

4.4 Diagnosis

Diagnosis of cardiac pathologies during dengue infection must be considered by clinicians, particularly in dengue-endemic areas. Patients suspected to have dengue fever must undergo routine hematological examination such as hemoglobin, total leucocyte counts, platelets, and hematocrit. Tourniquet test must be performed to rule out the any possiblity of severe dengue, i.e., DHF. Blood tests will not only aid to classify the severity of dengue infection but will also give clue of any cardiac involvement during infection. Chapter 1 describes various laboratory tests used in the diagnosis of dengue. Important blood tests performed for the diagnosis of dengue infection are enlisted below [36]:

- Detection of NS1 antigen of DENV is a rapid routine diagnostic test for DENV infection (usually becomes detectable in 1–2 days of dengue fever).
- IgM capture ELISA to detect IgM antibodies produced in response to DENV (becomes positive after 5 days and remains detectable up to 90 days).
- IgG ELISA to distinguish between primary and secondary dengue infection.
- For diagnosis of hepatic, renal, and cardiac involvement, a detailed blood workup should be done, such as LFTs, RFTs, and cardiac biomarkers.

4.4.1   Diagnostic Tests for Cardiac Involvement

As stated earlier, ECG abnormalities have been clearly demonstrated to provide evidence of myocardial involvement in dengue infection [3, 18, 37, 38]. Apart from echoradiography, radionuclide ventriculography is also used to assess cardiac function in patients with severe dengue [3]. Some common investigations for cardiac involvement in DENV infection include:

- Daily BP charting to monitor irregularities in blood pressure.
- ECG monitoring for the detection of any ECG abnormality as stated previously. If ECG abnormalities are detected, a repeat ECG is to be conducted on a daily basis to monitor ongoing cardiac injury.
- Pulse chart is to be maintained to detect any rate and rhythm abnormality.
- Cardiac enzymes (such as CK-MB, troponin 1, troponin 2, etc.) monitoring for the detection of cardiac insult.

4.4.2   Cardiac Biomarkers in Dengue

The monitoring of cardiac biomarkers is another important tool for the early identification of cardiac injury during the course of DVI. Several cardiac biomarkers detected in cardiac involvement include myoglobin, creatine kinase-muscle brain-type (CK-MB), N-terminal pro-brain natriuretic peptide, heart-type fatty acid-binding protein, troponins 1 and 2, and troponin T [39].

4.4.3   Histopathological Findings

Pleural effusions and ascites are seen in the chest and abdominal cavities at autopsy. Macroscopic and microscopic evidence of bleeding in muscles and internal organs is also observed in florid myocarditis [40]. The primary histopathological features are described below [23, 40, 41]:

- Interstitial edema with inflammatory cell infiltration of mainly fibroblasts, lymphomononuclear cells, and macrophage-type cells.
- Neutrophils can be seen in association with mononuclear cells during myocytolytic necrosis and necrosis of myocardial fibers.
- Dilated and flabby heart.
- Evidence of pericarditis.
- On electron microscopy, clustered virus particles are seen in diffuse foci of cardiomyocytes and interstitial space causing dissolution of myofilaments.
- Immunohistochemistry of virus particles in myocardial tissues reveals markedly stained mononuclear cells, while intracytoplasmic granular staining within some cardiomyocytes is also seen.

Apart from the histopathological changes in the heart, significant changes have also been observed in other organs, such as the lungs, liver, brain, and spleen. Major pulmonary changes include septal congestion, pulmonary hemorrhage, and diffuse alveolar damage, while necrosis of the liver can also be observed among patients.

4.5 Management

Cardiac manifestations suggestive of cardiac injury lack both sensitivity and specificity. Usually a cardiac insult in dengue infection is acute and transient, and there are no special guidelines available for the management. In most of the patients with DENV infection, myocarditis remains asymptomatic, and its management or treatment in the absence of clinical symptoms is unnecessary. ECG abnormalities provide a clear idea of myocarditis and should be monitored regularly in patients undergoing severe DENV infection [36].

The aim of the management is to provide a symptomatic care or supportive care to maintain hemodynamic stability. Supportive care includes maintenance of optimal intravascular blood volume, ionotropic support, and use of diuretics where necessary [22]. On the other hand, care should be taken to avoid iatrogenic fluid overload [42]. Although the current guidelines do not suggest the use of corticosteroids or immunoglobulins for the treatment of severe dengue [43], a case indicating a rapid recovery of child with myocarditis with IV administration of methyl prednisolone has been reported in the literature [44].

The role of anti-arrhythmics in the treatment of atrial fibrillation (AF) caused by dengue has not been clearly defined. Few studies have supported the use of anti-arrhythmics in non-self-limiting atrial fibrillation. However, the use of calcium channel blockers and beta-blockers in the management of AF caused by DENV infection is controversial due to co-existing hypotension [31]. Features such as AV dissociation, premature ventricular complexes, wall hypokinesia, and nonspecific ST–T changes are acute in nature and subside within 4–8 weeks of onset. It must be noted that strict monitoring and vigorous management to ensure hemodynamic stability are the mainstay of management.

References

1. Naresh G, Kulkarni AV, Sinha N, Jhamb N, Gulati S. Dengue hemorrhagic fever complicated with encephalopathy and myocarditis: a case report. J Commun Dis. 2008;40(3):223–4.
2. Gupta N, Kulkarni AV, Sinha N, Jhamb R, Gulati S. Dengue hemorrhagic fever complicated with encephalopathy and myocarditis. J Commun Dis. 2010;42(4):297–9.
3. Wali JP, Biswas A, Chandra S, Malhotra A, Aggarwal P, Handa R, et al. Cardiac involvement in dengue Haemorrhagic fever. Int J Cardiol. 1998;64(1):31–6.
4. Kularatne SA, Pathirage MM, Medagama UA, Gunasena S, Gunasekara MB. Myocarditis in three patients with dengue virus type DEN 3 infection. Ceylon Med J. 2006;51(2):75–6.
5. Guzman MG, Alvarez M, Rodriguez R, Rosario D, Vazquez S, Vald s L, et al. Fatal dengue hemorrhagic fever in Cuba, 1997. Int J Infect Dis. 1999;3(3):130–5.
6. Songco RS, Hayes CG, Leus CD, Manaloto CO. Dengue fever/dengue haemorrhagic fever in Filipino children: clinical experience during the 1983–1984 epidemic. Southeast Asian J Trop Med Public Health. 1987;18(3):284–90.
7. Hober D, Poli L, Roblin B, Gestas P, Chungue E, Granic G, et al. Serum levels of tumor necrosis factor-alpha (TNF-alpha), interleukin-6 (IL-6), and interleukin-1 beta (IL-1 beta) in dengue-infected patients. Am J Trop Med Hyg. 1993;48(3):324–31.
8. Hober D, Delannoy AS, Benyoucef S, De Groote D, Wattre P. High levels of sTNFR p75 and TNF alpha in dengue-infected patients. Microbiol Immunol. 1996;40(8):569–73.
9. Chen RF, Yang KD, Wang L, Liu JW, Chiu CC, Cheng JT. Different clinical and laboratory manifestations between dengue haemorrhagic fever and dengue fever with bleeding tendency. Trans R Soc Trop Med Hyg. 2007;101(11):1106–13.
10. Chen RF, Liu JW, Yeh WT, Wang L, Chang JC, Yu HR, et al. Altered T helper 1 reaction but not increase of virus load in patients with dengue hemorrhagic fever. FEMS Immunol Med Microbiol. 2005;44(1):43–50.
11. Dhawan R, Khanna M, Chaturvedi UC, Mathur A. Effect of dengue virus-induced cytotoxin on capillary permeability. J Exp Pathol (Oxford). 1990;71(1):83–8.
12. Matsumori A, Sasayama S. Immunomodulating agents for the management of heart failure with myocarditis and cardiomyopathy—lessons from animal experiments. Eur Heart J. 1995;16(Suppl O):140–3.
13. Kuhl U, Noutsias M, Schultheiss HP. Immunohistochemistry in dilated cardiomyopathy. Eur Heart J. 1995;16(Suppl O):100–6.
14. Kasim YA, Anky Tri Rini KE, Sumarmo SP. Hyperventilation in children with dengue hemorrhagic fever (DHF). Paediatr Indones. 1991;31(9–10):245–52.
15. Sangle SA, Dasgupta A, Ratnalikar SD, Kulkarni RV. Dengue myositis and myocarditis. Neurol India. 2010;58(4):598–9.
16. Salgado DM, Eltit JM, Mansfield K, Panqueba C, Castro D, Vega MR, et al. Heart and skeletal muscle are targets of dengue virus infection. Pediatr Infect Dis J. 2010;29(3):238–42.
17. Yacoub S, Wertheim H, Simmons CP, Screaton G, Wills B. Cardiovascular manifestations of the emerging dengue pandemic. Nat Rev Cardiol. 2014;11(6):335–45.
18. Khongphatthanayothin A, Lertsapcharoen P, Supachokchaiwattana P, La-Orkhun V, Khumtonvong A, Boonlarptaveechoke C, et al. Myocardial depression in dengue hemorrhagic fever: prevalence and clinical description. Pediatr Crit Care Med. 2007;8(6):524–9.
19. Kabra SK, Juneja R, Madhulika, Jain Y, Singhal T, Dar L, et al. Myocardial dysfunction in children with dengue haemorrhagic fever. Natl Med J India. 1998;11(2):59–61.
20. Nimmannitya S, Thisyakorn U, Hemsrichart V. Dengue haemorrhagic fever with unusual manifestations. Southeast Asian J Trop Med Public Health. 1987;18(3):398–406.
21. Promphan W, Sopontammarak S, Pruekprasert P, Kajornwattanakul W, Kongpattanayothin A. Dengue myocarditis. Southeast Asian J Trop Med Public Health. 2004;35(3):611–3.
22. Lee IK, Lee WH, Liu JW, Yang KD. Acute myocarditis in dengue hemorrhagic fever: a case report and review of cardiac complications in dengue-affected patients. Int J Infect Dis. 2010;14(10):e919–22.
23. Miranda CH, Borges MC, Matsuno AK, Vilar FC, Gali LG, Volpe GJ, et al. Evaluation of cardiac involvement during dengue viral infection. Clin Infect Dis. 2013;57(6):812–9.

24. Kularatne SA, Pathirage MM, Kumarasiri PV, Gunasena S, Mahindawanse SI. Cardiac complications of a dengue fever outbreak in Sri Lanka, 2005. Trans R Soc Trop Med Hyg. 2007;101(8):804–8.
25. Lateef A, Fisher DA, Tambyah PA. Dengue and relative bradycardia. Emerg Infect Dis. 2007;13(4):650–1.
26. Kaushik JS, Gupta P, Rajpal S, Bhatt S. Spontaneous resolution of sinoatrial exit block and atrioventricular dissociation in a child with dengue fever. Singap Med J. 2010;51(9):e146–8.
27. Khongphatthallayothin A, Chotivitayatarakorn P, Somchit S, Mitprasart A, Sakolsattayadorn S, Thisyakorn C. Morbitz type I second degree AV block during recovery from dengue hemorrhagic fever. Southeast Asian J Trop Med Public Health. 2000;31(4):642–5.
28. Kohli U, Sahu J, Lodha R, Agarwal N, Ray R. Invasive nosocomial aspergillosis associated with heart failure and complete heart block following recovery from dengue shock syndrome. Pediatr Crit Care Med. 2007;8(4):389–91.
29. Silva FTM, Silva Junior GBD, Benevides AN, Daher EDF. Atrial flutter complicating severe leptospirosis: a case report. Rev Soc Bras Med Trop. 2013;46:246–8.
30. Horta Veloso H, Ferreira Junior JA, Braga de Paiva JM, Faria Honorio J, Junqueira Bellei NC, Vicenzo de Paola AA. Acute atrial fibrillation during dengue hemorrhagic fever. Braz J Infect Dis. 2003;7(6):418–22.
31. Mahmod M, Darul ND, Mokhtar I, Nor NM, Anshar FM, Maskon O. Atrial fibrillation as a complication of dengue hemorrhagic fever: non-self-limiting manifestation. Int J Infect Dis. 2009;13(5):e316–8.
32. Chuah SK. Transient ventricular arrhythmia as a cardiac manifestation in dengue haemorrhagic fever—a case report. Singap Med J. 1987;28(6):569–72.
33. La-Orkhun V, Supachokchaiwattana P, Lertsapcharoen P, Khongphatthanayothin A. Spectrum of cardiac rhythm abnormalities and heart rate variability during the convalescent stage of dengue virus infection: a Holter study. Ann Trop Paediatr. 2011;31(2):123–8.
34. Lee CH, Teo C, Low AF. Fulminant dengue myocarditis masquerading as acute myocardial infarction. Int J Cardiol. 2009;136(3):e69–71.
35. Salgado DM, Panqueba CA, Castro D, Vega MR, Rodriguez JA. [Myocarditis in children affected by dengue hemorrhagic fever in a teaching hospital in Colombia]. Rev Salud Publica (Bogota). 2009;11(4):591–600.
36. Wiwanitkit V. Dengue fever: diagnosis and treatment. Expert review of anti-infective therapy. 2010;8(7):841–5.
37. Khongphatthanayothin A, Suesaowalak M, Muangmingsook S, Bhattarakosol P, Pancharoen C. Hemodynamic profiles of patients with dengue hemorrhagic fever during toxic stage: an echocardiographic study. Intensive Care Med. 2003;29(4):570–4.
38. Miranda CH, Borges Mde C, Matsuno AK, Vilar FC, Gali LG, Volpe GJ, et al. Evaluation of cardiac involvement during dengue viral infection. Clin Infect Dis. 2013;57(6):812–9.
39. Wichmann D, Kularatne S, Ehrhardt S, Wijesinghe S, Brattig NW, Abel W, et al. Cardiac involvement in dengue virus infections during the 2004/2005 dengue fever season in Sri Lanka. Southeast Asian J Trop Med Public Health. 2009;40(4):727–30.
40. Weerakoon KG, Kularatne SA, Edussuriya DH, Kodikara SK, Gunatilake LP, Pinto VG, et al. Histopathological diagnosis of myocarditis in a dengue outbreak in Sri Lanka, 2009. BMC Res Notes. 2011;4:268.
41. Miranda CH, de Carvalho Borges M, Schmidt A, Pazin-Filho A, Rossi MA, Ramos SG, et al. A case presentation of a fatal dengue myocarditis showing evidence for dengue virus-induced lesion. Eur Heart J Acute Cardiovasc Care. 2013;2(2):127–30.
42. Seppelt IM, Orde SR. Why guess when you can see? Heart function and fluid management in dengue shock. Crit Care Med. 2012;40(2):675–6.
43. Rajapakse S, Rodrigo C, Rajapakse A. Treatment of dengue fever. Infect Drug Resist. 2012;5:103–12.
44. Premaratna R, Rodrigo KM, Anuratha A, de Alwis VK, Perera UD, de Silva HJ. Repeated dengue shock syndrome and 'dengue myocarditis' responding dramatically to a single dose of methyl prednisolone. Int J Infect Dis. 2012;16(7):e565–9.

Dengue-Induced Pulmonary Complications

5

5.1 Lung Involvements in Dengue Infection

Acute respiratory distress syndrome (ARDS) is a major complication that occurs in severe forms of dengue viral infection (DVI). ARDS in pediatric ICU is known to be caused by DSS, particularly in dengue endemic areas. Dengue virus (DENV) antigen is found in alveolar cells during ARDS and causes increased vascular permeability in alveoli resulting in interstitial and alveolar edema [1].

5.1.1 Pathogenesis

DHF is associated with increased vascular permeability, thrombocytopenia, and hemorrhage. The functional change in the endothelium is responsible for the plasma leakage during DHF. However, vascular complications can recover rapidly without any serious squeal [2]. The major factors responsible for evolution to DHF are virulence of infecting virus, host immune system, and its intrinsic factors [3–5].

Virus replication primarily takes place in the lung epithelium and cancer cell lines during the course of DVI [6]. The fact that lungs are susceptible to dengue infection is supported by the presence of dengue virus particles in lungs cells, viral RNA synthesis in cell, and release of viral particles in the supernatants [6]. The order of efficiency of replication of DENV in lung cells is as follows: DENV-2 > DENV-3 > DENV-4 > DENV-1 [6].

The lung epithelial cells are possibly targeted by the DENV. Both IL-6 and RANTES play a pivotal role in the pathogenesis of dengue-associated pulmonary complications [6]. Existing data elaborated that IL-6 and RANTES expressions are elevated in DENV-2 infection in four out of six lung cancer cell lines, and these molecules are highly expressed in patients with severe disease (DHF/DSS) [6]. The overall pulmonary pathogenesis includes pleural effusion, increased vascular permeability, plasma leakage, and hemostasis abnormalities [1]. Figure 5.1 describes the diagrammatical illustration of dengue-induced lung injury.

© Springer Nature Singapore Pte Ltd. 2021
T. H. Mallhi et al., *Expanded Dengue Syndrome*,
https://doi.org/10.1007/978-981-15-7337-8_5

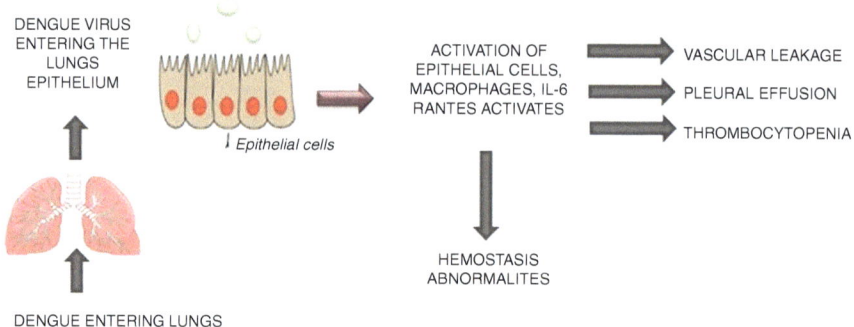

Fig. 5.1 Pathogenesis of dengue-induced lung injury

5.1.2 Clinical Manifestations

The severity of clinical manifestations of dengue-induced pulmonary disease varies from mild self-limiting illness to severe form of respiratory failure. The most common symptoms include:

1. Thoracic involvement is common as part of polyserositis during DHF. The severe lower respiratory tract involvement is rare. Since DF is febrile illness, it is less likely to be associated with respiratory symptoms [7–10].
2. ARDS in DHF and DSS is manifested as pleural effusion, pulmonary hemorrhage, pneumonia, and shock, which can result in severe dyspnea [11, 12].
3. Pleural effusion in DHF may be bloody or hemothorax and is a common feature of dyspnea [13, 14]. In patients with DF and non-dengue febrile illness, mild pleural effusions have been observed. The mild form of pleural effusion is not sufficient evidence for plasma leakage [15].
4. ARDS is characterized by respiratory depression, hypoxemia, radiographic infiltrates, and reduced lung compliance [16]. Increased alveolar–arterial oxygen gradient is commonly seen among these hypoxemic patients. Dengue patients having plasma leakage and undergoing fluid replacement have complications of noncardiac pulmonary edema [11, 17, 18]. Hence, confirmation of dengue infection should be ruled out in ARDS patients, particularly among patients residing in dengue epidemic areas [19].
5. Diffuse alveolar hemorrhage (DAH) resulting from bleeding into the acinar portion of the lung is also seen in severe dengue [20]. However, 40% of cases presented with DAH are without hemoptysis [20]. Patients having recognized pulmonary hemorrhage as hemoptysis are not frequently seen in DF [10, 21]. DAH in DHF is rare and scarcely reported in the literature [18, 21–23].

5.1.3 Diagnosis

Owing to the broad spectrum nonspecific clinical manifestations during the course of DVI, the diagnosis of dengue cannot solely rely on clinical symptoms. Hence, early laboratory confirmation followed by prompt intervention is pivotal and life-saving [24]. Diagnosis revolves around the detection of the virus particles and their components in patients. Moreover, patient's response to DENV is carried out during the diagnosis of DVI [23]. Diagnostic methods usually vary depending on the day of illness; as before day 5 of illness, dengue infection is diagnosed by isolation of dengue virus in cell culture, by nucleic acid amplification tests for detecting viral RNA, or by enzyme-linked immunosorbent assay (ELISA) for detection of viral antigens [23]. The confirmatory test for the febrile phase includes reverse-transcriptase polymerase chain reaction (RT-PCR), ELISA, or lateral-flow rapid test [24]. Immunoglobulin M (IgM) is considered to be a confirmatory finding and is required to confirm a presumptive diagnosis [25]. The detailed description of DVI diagnosis is described in Chap. 1.

5.1.3.1 Molecular Diagnosis
RT-PCR is an important diagnostic test for detection of dengue infection during the early phase [26]. RT-PCR is highly sensitive compared to virus isolation and allows rapid detection of dengue infections using minute quantities of virus and easy detection of the serotype circulating in blood [27].

5.1.3.2 Differential Diagnosis
In immunocompromised patients, different co-infections of various pathogens with DVI are challenging. Infectious diseases such as influenza A, leptospirosis, malaria, and hantavirus pulmonary syndrome (HPS) should be considered during the differential diagnosis. For detection of influenza virus in respiratory specimens, several laboratory tests are used including real-time RT-PCR. However, the diagnosis of leptospirosis is based on clinical findings [28–30]. The diagnosis of malaria should be considered as a possible cause of respiratory failure and must be ruled out during the diagnostic workup. Radiographic and CT findings in cases with malaria are consistent with noncardiogenic pulmonary edema. Parasites may be detected in peripheral blood smears [28–30].

5.1.3.3 Histopathology
Many histological evidences of lung involvement in DVI have been reported. This includes the presence of viral antigens in lung tissue and macrophage and lung endothelial and epithelial cell infection by virus [31, 32]. The presence of inflammatory cells in lung tissue, nuclear debris within alveolar spaces, and congestion of the vessels of alveolar wall have also been observed [11, 14, 18, 21, 22, 33–35]. Viral

antigens are also detected inside macrophages and endothelial cells [31]. The presence of interstitial inflammation and hemorrhage along with alveolar fluid, protein (including fibrin), and lung hemorrhage are the histopathological findings associated with fatal cases of dengue [36]. The most histological studies of lungs in patients with DF showed interstitial pneumonia in conjunction with vascular congestion. Other findings include increased number of alveolar macrophages along with recruiting of platelets, mononuclear, and polymorphonuclear cells [37]. On necropsy of human lung tissue, similar injuries have been observed in dengue fatal cases [38]. Viral replication was observed in alveolar macrophages of mice infected with DVI. Virus-like particles have been observed inside vesicles, Golgi complex, and rough endoplasmic reticulum, suggesting the viral replication [37].

5.1.3.4 Radiographic Findings

Among the most common abnormalities observed in chest CT, pleural effusion is the major finding [13]. Ground-glass opacity (GGO) and lung consolidation are other common findings of lung parenchymal involvement along with interlobular septal thickening and airspace nodules with no specific axial distribution [13]. On CT, acute phase corresponds to GGO without major interlobular septal wall thickening, whereas in the subacute phase, inter- and intralobular septal wall thickening develops, typically within 48 h. Acute airspace opacities and septal thickening are usually resolved within 2 weeks in a monophasic episode of pulmonary hemorrhage [13]. In pulmonary hemorrhage syndrome associated with DVI, extensive consolidation and diffused GGO in lungs have been reported in recent studies [13, 22]. These findings are consistent with DAH but are nonspecific [20].

5.1.3.5 Pathological Findings

Severe dengue is presented as an infection of many organs, and the lungs are commonly affected [19]. In severe cases of dengue, massive lung involvement usually showing lung hemorrhage is associated with fatal infections and shock [13]. The autopsy studies of dengue cases indicated pulmonary pathological findings as described below [32]:

- Infiltration with mononuclear cells
- Hyperplasia involving alveolar macrophages
- Hyaline membrane formation
- Hypertrophy of type II pneumocytes

In ARDS, mainly neutrophil recruitment in inflammation is usually seen, while mononuclear infiltrates have been associated in various dengue cases [32].

DENV antigens and viral replication is found in type II pneumocytes and pulmonary vascular endothelial cells [32]. Furthermore, in severe dengue acute DAH, septal hemorrhage, alveolar congestion, pleural effusion, and dilatation of subpleural lymphatic spaces are also seen [17–19, 22].

5.1.4   Management of Dengue-Induced Lung Injury

There is no specific treatment for the dengue-induced lung injury, but careful clinical management frequently could save the lives of patients. There is often a delay in early recognition and initiation of appropriate supportive therapy, which results in increased morbidity and mortality in dengue cases. Fluid administration plays a major role in avoiding respiratory depression secondary to other symptoms of lungs like massive pleural effusions or pulmonary edema [39]. Prolonged hospitalization is required when patients develop massive pleural effusions or ascites. Pleural effusion is usually detected between 5 and 7 days of illness with ultrasonography in great number of patients with dengue fever [40].

To avoid risk due to various forms of dengue fever, differential diagnosis should be done, and then proper supportive therapy should be given [22]. Also, various interactions between serotypes of DENV and their effects on lung tissue should be considered, as this would help for better diagnosis and treatment of lung complications [22, 40].

Frequent assessment of fluid and electrolyte balance and sufficient fluid administration are vital. Vital signs and packed cell volume should be monitored every 1–2 and 4–6 h, respectively. However, the rate at which the fluid is administered depends on degree of plasma leakage and body [41]. Fluid requirement in DHF is calculated (according to Halliday and Segar formula) as follows [42]:

- <10 kg body weight: 100 ml/kg
- 10–20 kg body weight: 1000 ml + 50 ml for each kg in excess of 10 kg
- >20 kg body weight: 1500 ml + 20 ml for each kg in excess of 20 kg

Various types of fluid can be used for The management of dengue-induced lung injury. The WHO recommend crystalloid solutions, while there are some studies that suggest to use colloidal solution (dextran 70 or 3% gelatin) at first and then crystalloid solutions [42]. In patients that develop serious hemorrhagic symptoms or have severe thrombocytopenia, platelet transfusions may be administered [43]. When platelet transfusions are given, a reduction in active bleeding is seen. Moreover, the degree of increase in circulating platelets is proportional to the amount of platelets infused [44].

In case of DSS, quick and sufficient fluid administration is required. The patient should be asked to lay down on a flat surface, and oxygen should be given. Vital signs and oxygen saturation should be monitored every 10–15 min. Intravenous fluid should be infused, while blood transfusions are administered after confirming match. Electrolyte abnormalities, hypoglycemia, metabolic acidosis, and disseminated intravascular coagulation in these patients can lead to massive bleeding. Prothrombin time should be checked, and blood transfusions (blood, fresh frozen plasma, and platelet transfusions) should be administered in patients who develop intravascular coagulation. Ideal management of fluids in this case includes both crystalloids and colloids (including albumin) [45]. Though the incidence of pulmonary manifestations is high among the complicated cases of dengue fever (DHF and DSS), dengue-induced lung complications have satisfactory prognosis with prompt and aggressive management. Moreover, respiratory manifestations can be used as an indicator of serious presentation for the DVI.

References

1. Mohamed NA, El-Raoof EA, Ibraheem HA. Respiratory manifestations of dengue fever in Taiz-Yemen. Egypt J Chest Dis Tuberc. 2013;62(2):319–23.
2. Libraty DH, Endy TP, Houng HS, Green S, Kalayanarooj S, Suntayakorn S, et al. Differing influences of virus burden and immune activation on disease severity in secondary dengue-3 virus infections. J Infect Dis. 2002;185(9):1213–21.
3. Kliks SC, Nisalak A, Brandt WE, Wahl L, Burke DS. Antibody-dependent enhancement of dengue virus growth in human monocytes as a risk factor for dengue hemorrhagic fever. Am J Trop Med Hyg. 1989;40(4):444–51.
4. Rico-Hesse R, Harrison LM, Salas RA, Tovar D, Nisalak A, Ramos C, et al. Origins of dengue type 2 viruses associated with increased pathogenicity in the Americas. Virology. 1997;230(2):244–51.
5. Stephens HA. HLA and other gene associations with dengue disease severity. Curr Top Microbiol Immunol. 2010;338:99–114.
6. Lee YR, Su CY, Chow NH, Lai WW, Lei HY, Chang CL, et al. Dengue viruses can infect human primary lung epithelia as well as lung carcinoma cells, and can also induce the secretion of IL-6 and RANTES. Virus Res. 2007;126(1–2):216–25.
7. Potts JA, Rothman AL. Clinical and laboratory features that distinguish dengue from other febrile illnesses in endemic populations. Tropical Med Int Health. 2008;13(11):1328–40.
8. Mustafa B, Hani AW, Chem YK, Mariam M, Khairul AH, Abdul Rasid K, et al. Epidemiological and clinical features of dengue versus other acute febrile illnesses amongst patients seen at government polyclinics. Med J Malaysia. 2010;65(4):291–6.
9. Halsey ES, Marks MA, Gotuzzo E, Fiestas V, Suarez L, Vargas J, et al. Correlation of serotype-specific dengue virus infection with clinical manifestations. PLoS Negl Trop Dis. 2012;6(5):e1638.
10. Hayes CG, Manaloto CR, Gonzales A, Ranoa CP. Dengue infections in the Philippines: clinical and virological findings in 517 hospitalized patients. Am J Trop Med Hyg. 1988;39(1):110–6.
11. Sen MK, Ojha UC, Chakrabarti S, Suri JC. Dengue hemorrhagic fever (DHF) presenting with ARDS. Indian J Chest Dis Allied Sci. 1999;41(2):115–9.
12. Nelson ER. Hemorrhagic fever in children in Thailand: report of 69 cases. J Pediatr. 1960;56(1):101–8.
13. Rodrigues RS, Brum ALG, Paes MV, Póvoa TF, Basilio-de-Oliveira CA, Marchiori E, et al. Lung in dengue: computed tomography findings. PLoS One. 2014;9(5):e96313.
14. Karanth SS, Gupta A, Prabhu M. Unilateral massive hemothorax in dengue hemorrhagic fever: a unique presentation. Asian Pac J Trop Med. 2012;5(9):753–4.
15. Srikiatkhachorn A, Krautrachue A, Ratanaprakarn W, Wongtapradit L, Nithipanya N, Kalayanarooj S, et al. Natural history of plasma leakage in dengue hemorrhagic fever: a serial ultrasonographic study. Pediatr Infect Dis J. 2007;26(4):283–90. discussion 91-2
16. Devarajan TV, Prashant PS, Mani AK, Victor SM, Khan PS. Dengue with ARDS. J Indian Acad Clin Med. 2008;9:146–9.
17. Wang CC, Liu SF, Liao SC, Lee IK, Liu JW, Lin AS, et al. Acute respiratory failure in adult patients with dengue virus infection. Am J Trop Med Hyg. 2007;77(1):151–8.

18. Setlik RF, Ouellette D, Morgan J, McAllister CK, Dorsey D, Agan BK, et al. Pulmonary hemorrhage syndrome associated with an autochthonous case of dengue hemorrhagic fever. South Med J. 2004;97(7):688–91.
19. Idirisinghe KAP. Histopathological study of dengue Haemorrhagic fever. J Diagn Pathol. 2014;8(1):50–8.
20. de Prost N, Parrot A, Cuquemelle E, Picard C, Antoine M, Fleury-Feith J, et al. Diffuse alveolar hemorrhage in immunocompetent patients: etiologies and prognosis revisited. Respir Med. 2012;106(7):1021–32.
21. Liam CK, Yap BH, Lam SK. Dengue fever complicated by pulmonary haemorrhage manifesting as haemoptysis. J Trop Med Hyg. 1993;96(3):197–200.
22. Marchiori E, Ferreira JLN, Bittencourt CN, de Araújo Neto CA, Zanetti G, Mano CM, et al. Pulmonary hemorrhage syndrome associated with dengue fever, high-resolution computed tomography findings: a case report. Orphanet J Rare Dis. 2009;4:8.
23. Wilder-Smith A, Ooi E-E, Horstick O, Wills B. Dengue. Lancet. 2019;393(10169):350–63.
24. Simmons CP, Farrar JJ, van Vinh Chau N, Wills B. Dengue. N Engl J Med. 2012;366(15):1423–32.
25. Mallhi TH, Khan AH, Adnan AS, Sarriff A, Khan YH, Jummaat F. Clinico-laboratory spectrum of dengue viral infection and risk factors associated with dengue hemorrhagic fever: a retrospective study. BMC Infect Dis. 2015;15(1):399.
26. Velathanthiri N, Fernando R, Fernando S. Development of a polymerase chain reaction (PCR) for the detection of dengue virus and its sero types. Abstract presented at the Sri Lanka College of Microbiologists annual sessions. 2002.
27. De Paula SO, Pires RJ, Corrêa JAT, Assumpção SR, Costa ML, Lima DM, et al. The use of reverse transcription-polymerase chain reaction (RT-PCR) for the rapid detection and identification of dengue virus in an endemic region: a validation study. Trans R Soc Trop Med Hyg. 2002;96(3):266–9.
28. Aye KS, Charngkaew K, Win N, Wai KZ, Moe K, Punyadee N, et al. Pathologic highlights of dengue hemorrhagic fever in 13 autopsy cases from Myanmar. Hum Pathol. 2014;45(6):1221–33.
29. Marchiori E, Müller NL. Leptospirosis of the lung: high-resolution computed tomography findings in five patients. J Thorac Imaging. 2002;17(2):151–3.
30. Marchiori E, Lourenço S, Setúbal S, Zanetti G, Gasparetto TD, Hochhegger B. Clinical and imaging manifestations of hemorrhagic pulmonary leptospirosis: a state-of-the-art review. Lung. 2011;189(1):1–9.
31. Jessie K, Fong MY, Devi S, Lam SK, Wong KT. Localization of dengue virus in naturally infected human tissues, by immunohistochemistry and in situ hybridization. J Infect Dis. 2004;189(8):1411–8.
32. Póvoa TF, Alves AMB, Oliveira CAB, Nuovo GJ, Chagas VLA, Paes MV. The pathology of severe dengue in multiple organs of human fatal cases: histopathology, ultrastructure and virus replication. PLoS One. 2014;9(4):e83386.
33. Lum LC, Thong MK, Cheah YK, Lam SK. Dengue-associated adult respiratory distress syndrome. Ann Trop Paediatr. 1995;15(4):335–9.
34. Sharma SK, Gupta BS, Devpura G, Agarwal A, Anand S. Pulmonary haemorrhage syndrome associated with dengue haemorrhagic fever. J Assoc Physicians India. 2007;55:729–30.
35. Kumar N, Gadpayle AK, Trisal D. Atypical respiratory complications of dengue fever. Asian Pac J Trop Med. 2013;6(10):839–40.
36. Mahajan SN, Rathi NP, Acharya S. ARDS in dengue infection—a case Series. Indian J Med Healthc. 2013;2(2):235–7.
37. Barreto DF, Takiya CM, Schatzmayr HG, Nogueira RM, da Costa Farias-Filho J, Barth OM. Histopathological and ultrastructural aspects of mice lungs experimentally infected with dengue virus serotype 2. Mem Inst Oswaldo Cruz. 2007;102(2):175–82.
38. Miagostovich MP, Ramos RG, Nicol AF, Nogueira RM, Cuzzi-Maya T, Oliveira AV, et al. Retrospective study on dengue fatal cases. Clin Neuropathol. 1997;16(4):204–8.
39. Lum L, Ng CJ, Khoo EM. Managing dengue fever in primary care: a practical approach. Malays Fam Physician. 2014;9(2):2–10.

40. Zaki SA. Pleural effusion and ultrasonography in dengue Fever. Indian J Community Med. 2011;36(2):163.
41. Holliday MA, Segar WE. The maintenance need for water in parenteral fluid therapy. Pediatrics. 1957;19(5):823–32.
42. Wills B. Volume replacement in dengue shock syndrome. Dengue Bulletin. 2001;25:50–55.
43. Chuansumrit A, Phimolthares V, Tardtong P, Tapaneya-Olarn C, Tapaneya-Olarn W, Kowsathit P, et al. Transfusion requirements in patients with dengue hemorrhagic fever. Southeast Asian J Trop Med Public Health. 2000;31(1):10–4.
44. Isarangkura P, Tuchinda S. The behavior of transfused platelets in dengue hemorrhagic fever. Southeast Asian J Trop Med Public Health. 1993;24:222–4.
45. Soni A, Chugh K, Sachdev A, Gupta D. Management of dengue fever in ICU. Indian J Pediatr. 2001;68(11):1051–5.

Dengue-Induced Neurological Complications

6

6.1 Neurological Involvements in Dengue Infection

The World Health Organization (WHO) in its recent guidelines (2009) includes central nervous system (CNS) involvement in the definition of severe dengue [1, 2]. However, detailed description of neurological complications is not provided in these guidelines. The frequency and clinical spectrum of these manifestations are less known. From the time dengue was recognized as a clinical entity, neurological complications of the disease have been described [3–5]. The first case of neurological involvement was reported in 1976 as an atypical manifestation of dengue infection [6]. The prevalence rates of neurological disorders varied from 0.5 to 20% in recent years. These complications have been reported in all age groups and in all types of dengue infection, i.e., DF, DHF, and DSS of WHO 1997 classification and dengue with and without warning signs and severe dengue according to WHO 2009 criterion [7]. Neurological complications have been reported in 25 countries across all continents [8].

The reported time of onset of neurological symptoms during the course of dengue infection is 3–7 days from the start of fever [9]. Neurological manifestations as initial symptoms are rarely reported in the literature [10]. Factors that might contribute to the neuropathies may include prolonged shock, hepatic failure, intracranial bleeding, or hyponatremia [3]. It must be noted that abnormal neurological manifestations during the course of dengue infection might be due to encephalopathy rather than encephalitis. Dengue virus (DENV)-associated neurotropism was extensively established in the late 1990s resulting in an increased number of reports. Since 1990, numerous studies reported the isolated virus from cerebro spinal fluid (CSF) or brain tissues [7].

© Springer Nature Singapore Pte Ltd. 2021
T. H. Mallhi et al., *Expanded Dengue Syndrome*,
https://doi.org/10.1007/978-981-15-7337-8_6

6.1.1 Clinical Spectrum of Dengue-Induced Neurological Complications

Most of the neurological complications of dengue infection are reported through isolated case reports or small case series. These studies presented diverse spectrum of CNS involvements which preclude classifying neurological manifestations in clinical practice. Previously, dengue-induced neurological complications were categorized into three groups. This classification is based on the pathogenesis and includes:

1. Neurological abnormalities associated with metabolic disturbances: encephalopathy
2. Neurological involvements caused by viral invasion: encephalitis, meningitis, myositis, and myelitis
3. Neurological involvements due to autoimmune reactions

Autoimmune reactions cause a wide range of neurological anomalies including acute disseminated encephalomyelitis, neuromyelitis optica, optic neuritis, neuritis brachialis, myelitis, post-infectious encephalopathy, and Guillain–Barré syndrome [8, 11].

In the recent years, neurological involvements have been extended to central nervous system and eyes, associated peripheral nervous system (PNS) syndromes, and convalescent or post-dengue immune-mediated syndromes [12, 13]. Of these, meningitis, encephalitis, encephalopathy, and myelitis are the most important and well-studied neuroinvasive complications associated with DVI. It is important to note that DENV-associated meningitis is more frequent among children. Meningitis caused by other viral infections does not frequently occur in children. However, clinical manifestations of dengue-induced meningitis are similar to other viral meningitis [13].

There is a wide diversity in the clinical spectrum of neurological complications which is primarily related to the location of the lesions. Following is the list of frequent neurological presentations among patients with acute dengue [14].

- Headache
- Mood changes/irritability
- Sleep disturbances/insomnia
- Seizures
- Encephalopathy
- Stroke
- Focal neurological deficit associated with encephalitis
- Altered consciousness

Dengue patients with myelitis and myositis may present with symptoms related to motor deficit. However, deficit can also occur during post-dengue stage among patients with encephalomyelitis, neuromyelitis optica, polyradiculoneuritis, mono-neuropathy, and polyneuropathy [14].

Unfortunately, the true incidence of dengue-induced encephalopathy is not known. According to a case–control study conducted in Vietnam, the prevalence of dengue-induced encephalopathy accounted for 0.5% among patients with confirmatory diagnosis of DHF [15]. In another study conducted on laboratory-confirmed Thai children, neurological symptoms were present in 5.4% of cases. Of these, almost 50% children were presented with encephalopathy [16].

6.1.2   Pathogenesis of Dengue-Induced Neurological Complications

The mechanisms of neurological involvements during the course of DVI are assumed to be related to the specific type of neurological disease. However, viral and host factors play a pivotal role in the pathogenesis of disease. As described earlier, neuropathogenesis might be attributed to the direct viral invasion of the CNS [17], autoimmune reactions, and metabolic disturbances or alterations [18, 19]. Previously, dengue virus (DENV) was not considered as non-neurotropic. However, growing body of evidences has changed the concept and established neurotropic feature of DENV. The evidence of DENV in the CNS has already been described around 25 years ago [20, 21]. Moreover, it has been demonstrated that DENV damages blood–brain barrier (BBB) during infection in experimental animal models, indicating viral invasion [22]. Neurological complications according to the pathogenesis are described in Table 6.1. Initially DENV neurotropism in the human host was considered as opportunistic feature [24]. However, recent data establishes the notion that dengue virus is highly neurotropic in *Aedes aegypti* and is direct neurovirulent in humans [8, 25]. The neurological examinations of the CNS have detected viral proteins, ribonucleic acid (RNA), and immunoglobulins [26], indicating the DENV can actively enter the CNS [27]. Immunoreactive neurons, astrocytes, microglia, and endothelial cells have also been detected in cerebral tissues of a fatal case with dengue hemorrhagic fever [24]. Existing literature indicate that DENV-2 and DENV-3 are two common serotypes predominantly involved in the neurological complications [28, 29].

Table 6.1 Neurological complications in dengue according to pathogenesis

Metabolic disturbances	Viral invasion	Autoimmune reaction
Encephalopathy	Encephalitis	Acute disseminated encephalomyelitis
	Meningitis	Neuromyelitis optica
	Myositis	Optic neuritis
	Myelitis	Myelitis
		Post-infectious encephalopathy
		Guillain–Barré syndrome
		Neuritis brachialis

Sources: Table is adapted from reference [23] which is open access and does not require permission

6.1.3   Treatment and Prognosis of Dengue-Induced Neurological Complications

Due to the unavailability of licensed vaccine or specific treatments to prevent dengue or the associated neurological diseases, the treatment of these complications is tailored to the diagnosis [30, 31]. Most of the patients demonstrate benign evolution with spontaneous recovery. This type of disease pattern has been markedly observed among dengue patients having encephalitis or Guillain–Barré syndrome [32]. The prognostic and the clinical features of Guillain–Barré syndrome resemble to those reported for other infectious diseases. About 20–30% patients portend neurological squeal following the course of DVI. These include myelitis-related spastic paraparesis and urinary retention [17, 32, 33]. Dengue patients with encephalitis may experience mental confusion and personality alterations. Although case fatality rate due to dengue infection ranges from 3 to 5% [2], it may rise to 5–30% among patients with neurological involvements [16, 32–35]. Most of these mortality cases are associated with severe form of infection including DHF, DSS, or severe dengue.

6.1.4   Diagnosis of Dengue-Induced Neurological Complications

The diagnosis of neurological disease associated with DVI can be the same as used for the diagnosis of dengue infection itself such as positive dengue IgM, viral antigens, and virus RNA. However, these diagnostic methods are only sufficient for the patients experiencing acute neurological symptoms. Diagnosis of neurological manifestations is complex for oligosymptomatic or asymptomatic dengue patients. For such instances, hematological tests, cerebrospinal fluid analysis, and MR images are of great value. These tests not only provide the confirmatory diagnosis but also aid during differential diagnosis to exclude other possible causes of neurological disturbances. Dengue patients possessing neurological complications must undergo these diagnostic methods for vigilant monitoring and for better understanding of pathological mechanisms. All suspected cases must be subjected to routine laboratory investigations which may include:

- Hematologic tests
- Biochemical parameters
- Live function tests
- Tests for rheumatic diseases
- Tests for hepatitis B and C
- Test for human immunodeficiency virus-1 (HIV-1)

Since CSF analysis is of utmost importance for the definitive diagnosis of neurological disturbances, this analysis must include the following parameters:

- Total and specific cell count
- Protein concentration
- Glucose/lactate concentration

- A smear and culture for bacteria and fungi
- Albumin quotient (CSF/serum) for the assessment of functioning of blood–CSF barrier
- Detection of intrathecal synthesis of total IgG
- Measurement of specific antibodies against other viral diseases

Numerous viral diseases may contribute to neurological complications. These infections include syphilis, cytomegalovirus, Epstein–Barr, and herpes simplex viruses. CSF analysis-based differential diagnosis will tailor the appropriate management without adverse squeal [23].

6.2 Dengue-Induced Neurological Manifestations versus Japanese Encephalitis

Both DVI and Japanese encephalitis share similar neurological manifestations. It must be noted that several regions which are endemic for dengue viruses are also endemic for Japanese encephalitis virus. Antibodies in response to both infections are cross-reactive. Patients having encephalopathy with positive anti-flavivirus antibody in the CSF must be considered as candidate for diagnosis of Japanese encephalitis. The diagnostic tests for these two viruses are now in practice and widely used in endemic regions. However, available evidences suggest that neurological manifestations of dengue infection are likely to be recognized more often [17]. This can be evident from a study conducted in Thailand in which 4 out of 44 suspected Japanese encephalitis patients had confirmed dengue infection diagnosed by ELISA-based IgM detection [36].

6.3 Dengue Encephalopathy

Encephalopathy is a generalized term used to describe abnormalities in the functions and structure of the brain. Acute encephalopathy is most common neurological abnormalities present among dengue patients during their course of infection. Dengue encephalopathy is characterized by diminished level of consciousness. This altered consciousness is attributed to various precipitating factors. Following are the some important factors associated with diminished level of consciousness [33]:

- Prolonged shock
- Anoxia
- Cerebral edema
- Metabolic disturbances such as hyponatremia
- Systemic hemorrhages
- Cerebral hemorrhages
- Acute hepatic failure
- Acute kidney failure

Cognitive disorders, convulsions, and mood, personality, and behavior disorders are few primary symptoms of encephalopathy. Most of the cases of dengue encephalopathy are reported in children from developing countries. It is important to note that these cases do not show CSF abnormalities. Dengue encephalopathy is a deadly complication with associated mortality around 50% among affected cases [37].

6.3.1 Pathogenesis of Dengue Encephalopathy

Dengue encephalopathy has classically been thought to result from the multisystem derangement occurring in severe dengue with liver failure, shock, and coagulopathy, thereby causing cerebral insult. Encephalopathy in severe dengue such as DHF or DSS is triggered by various precursors as described below [8]:

- Brain edema
- Anoxia
- Hemorrhage
- Intense hyponatremia
- Liver failure
- Kidney failure
- Release of toxic substances
- Metabolic acidosis

Dengue viral neurotropism may result in direct viral encephalitis which may lead to encephalopathy. Neurotropic effect of virus as a cause of encephalopathy has been observed in a substantial number of cases [38].

It is crucial to differentiate encephalopathy and encephalitis that usually occur during DHF and DSS. There are several factors secondary to the infection which are potential determinants of encephalopathy and demonstrate no association with encephalitis. These factors must be taken into consideration during differential diagnosis and are described below [39]:

- Cerebral anoxia
- Shock
- Edema caused by liver failure
- Hemorrhages associated with low platelet counts
- Electrolyte disturbances

6.3.2 Clinical Manifestations of Dengue Encephalopathy

Dengue encephalopathy can be reflected by various neuro-cognitive manifestations. Following are the typical neuro-cognitive abnormalities presented among patients with dengue encephalopathy [8]:

- Reduced sensitivity
- Impaired cognitive abilities
- Seizures/convulsions
- Personality disorders
- Behavior disorders
- Acute mania
- Anxiety and depression
- Emotional liability
- Psychosis
- Agoraphobia

6.3.3 Diagnosis of Dengue Encephalopathy

CSF analyses, including measurements of protein, glucose, and cell count, are usually normal. However, sometimes CSF pleocytosis and high level of proteins may present among dengue patients [16]. Neuroimaging studies (computed tomography and/or magnetic resonance imaging (MRI) scan) may be normal or show diffuse cerebral edema, signal changes in involved regions, and extensive involvement of the bilateral cerebellar region, brainstem, and thalami along with peculiar rim enhancement [15, 35, 40].

6.3.4 Management of Dengue Encephalopathy

The treatment of dengue encephalopathy is primarily symptomatic with special care for maintenance of fluid and electrolyte imbalance. However, antiepileptics can be given to the patients [41]. The clinical outcomes of dengue-associated encephalopathy widely vary among cases and primarily depend on the causal factors. Though mortality associated with dengue encephalopathy is low but it can be high if supportive measures are not initiated in timely manners [42].

6.4 Dengue Encephalitis

Encephalitis is among the most common neurological manifestations of DVI. Dengue encephalitis is found in the three classical disease groups of dengue classification including DF, DHF, and DSS. Its frequency has been reported to range from 4.2 to 51% [21, 34, 43]. This wide disparity in the reported frequency is attributed to the predominant serotype DENV-2 and DENV-3 during epidemics, as both these serotypes are primarily associated with neurological involvements [23].

6.4.1   Pathogenesis of Dengue Encephalitis

Neurotropism associated with DENV and its ability to invade CNS resulted in an expanded clinical spectrum of encephalitis in recent studies. The neuropathogenesis of dengue encephalitis is primarily concerned with neurotropism, i.e., viral invasion. In vitro studies have demonstrated that mutant DENV-1 causes an extensive leptomeningitis and encephalitis in mice. It is hypothesized that mutant DENV can cross the blood–brain barrier due to neurotropism. Dengue virus neurotropism can also be evidenced by detection of intrathecal synthesis of specific antibodies in patients with dengue myelitis [44].

6.4.2   Clinical Manifestations of Dengue Encephalitis

The primary clinical manifestations of dengue encephalitis are seizures, altered consciousness, and headaches. Tetraparesis is also observed in the literature, particularly in severe cases [33]. Seizure is a typical clinical feature of neurological damage and is more common among patients with dengue encephalitis as compared to those with encephalopathy [45]. Unexpectedly, the prevalence of the typical symptoms of DVI such as myalgias, rash, bleeding, diarrhea, and joint or abdominal pain was only 50% among dengue encephalitis cases [9, 46]. Therefore, DENV would not ordinarily be suspected to be the cause of the neurological disease [27]. Dengue-associated encephalitis and encephalopathy are closely related to each other and most of the time indistinguishable. Therefore, acute liver failure (ALF), intracranial hemorrhage, and hypovolemic shock with metabolic deteriorations should rule out. CSF examinations should be considered on individual cases based on its safety and feasibility [8].

6.4.3   Diagnosis of Dengue Encephalitis

The diagnosis of dengue encephalitis requires careful consideration. The following criteria can be utilized to identify the cases of dengue-induced encephalitis [46]:

- Hyperthermia
- Acute signs of cerebral involvement: altered consciousness or personality, seizures, or focal neurological manifestations
- Presence of anti-dengue immunoglobulin M (IgM) in the serum and CSF
- Presence of dengue genomic material in the serum or CSF
- Exclusion of other potential or suspected triggers of viral encephalitis and encephalopathy

Computed tomography (CT) and magnetic resonance imaging (MRI) demonstrate widely diverse results. Hemorrhage, diffuse cerebral edema, and focal abnormalities might be present among patients. These abnormalities involve the globus pallidus, the hippocampus, the thalamus, and the internal capsule region of CNS. The lesions are hyper-intense as visualized by MRI [35]. CSF analysis may demonstrate inflammatory reaction, with lymphomononuclear pleocytosis and normal levels of glucose. However, normal CSF cellularity has been observed in 50% of cases with dengue encephalitis [43]. The absence of pleocytosis in CSF has been described in 5% of viral encephalitis cases. However, it can be speculated that this number is underestimated with regard to dengue infection [47]. In this context, the diagnosis of encephalitis should not be disregarded due to normal CSF cellularity [43].

Diagnostic evaluation of some patients with neurological symptoms demonstrates presence of DENV in CSF, but lacks evidence of its presence in the serum. These findings contradict the hypothesis that vascular leakage or rupture of the blood–brain barrier (BBB) is a pathogenic mechanism of dengue encephalitis. Detection of viral antigen in brain tissue, concomitant CSF pleocytosis, and viral RNA amplification in the CSF are some important evidences to support the invasive neurotropism of DENV [7]. The amplification of viral RNA can be seen in CSF during the acute infection [17]. Autopsy studies also support the DENV neurotropism. Moreover, viral antigens have been isolated from brain tissues of dengue fatal cases. Both immunohistochemistry and reverse transcriptase polymerase chain reaction assay (RT-PCR) have detected DENV-4 among DHF cases in the inferior olivary nucleus of medulla and in the granular layer of cerebellum. Immunoreactivity has been observed in neurons, astrocytes, microglia, and endothelial cells [24]. However, there is no specific neuroimaging findings suggestive of dengue encephalitis reported yet. The findings of brain MRI can be normal or may demonstrate some focal parenchymal abnormalities [15, 24]. Symmetric gyral edema and altered signal intensity involving bilateral temporal perisylvian regions, hippocampi, and cingulated gyri have been reported [48]. Evidences also suggest the involvement of the thalamus, pons, and bilateral cerebellum cortex. Postcontrast MRI has also shown occasional meningeal enhancement during the course of DVI [49].

6.4.4 Management of Dengue Encephalitis

There is no specific treatment of dengue encephalitis. Mostly symptomatic treatment is provided to the patients. The prognosis of dengue encephalitis is satisfactory, and minimal neurological deficit can be present on hospital discharge [50]. However, encephalitis may associate with high mortality among dengue patients. The outcome of dengue encephalitis is variable, with most patients recovering spontaneously. However, deaths have also been reported among patients with dengue encephalitis [7, 19, 51–53].

6.5 Dengue Meningitis

Meningitis refers to the inflammation of protective layers around the CNS called meninges. The prevalence of dengue-induced meningitis ranges from 24.4 to 30% in children [34]. The dengue meningitis rarely manifests in adults [43]. The clinical manifestations of dengue meningitis are similar to those reported for other types of viral meningitis [28].

6.5.1 Pathogenesis of Dengue Meningitis

Dengue-induced meningitis is attributed to the direct tissue lesion caused by the virus because of its neurotropicity, capillary hemorrhage, disseminated intravascular coagulation (DIC), and metabolic disorders [54].

6.5.2 Clinical Manifestations of Dengue Meningitis

Dengue patients with meningitis may present with fever, generalized or throbbing headache, neck pain, neck rigidity (nuchal rigidity), and vomiting. Dengue meningitis might cause migraine such as headaches with poor response to anti-migraine therapy and common analgesics [55].

6.5.3 Diagnosis of Dengue Meningitis

Since meningitis frequently occurs along with other viral infections, the testing of malaria, brucella, cytomegalovirus (CMV), Epstein–Barr virus (EBV), human immunodeficiency virus (HIV), and swine flu virus (H1N1) should be considered to exclude the other causes of meningitis. Diagnostic workup revolves around CSF examination. Immunoglobulin M has been identified in CSF [55]. Detection of DENV in CSF through PCR is another tool during diagnostic workup. Inflammatory CSF manifested by pleocytosis, hyperproteinorhachia, blood–CSF barrier dysfunction (albumin quotient $\geq 8 \times 10^{-3}$), and intrathecal synthesis of total IgG (IgG index ≥ 0.7 or oligoclonal IgG bands) is also an important characteristic of dengue meningitis [10, 56]. However, CSF cellularity, brain CT, and MRI scans can be normal among patients. Classical tests of meningitis including positive Kernig's sign, Brudzinski's sign, and nuchal rigidity should be carried out among suspected cases [10].

6.5.4 Management of Dengue Meningitis

There is no effective antiviral therapy to treat dengue meningitis and patients are managed symptomatically. Classical anti-migraine therapy has shown no or little response in pain management. However, tramadol and NSAIDs were proved partially effective [55]. Appropriate fluid resuscitation therapy has been evidenced with marked clinical improvements. However, full recovery is observed after few months among patients without any residual neurological deficit [28].

6.6   Dengue-Induced Transverse Myelitis

The term myelitis refers to inflammation of the spinal cord. This inflammation causes the damages to the nerve fibers which results in lose myelin sheath. Absence of the myelin sheath around the nerve fibers leads to decreased electrical conductivity in the CNS. In transverse myelitis (TM), the inflammation extends across the entire width of the spinal cord. When the inflammation affects part of the width of the spinal cord, the myelitis is referred to as partial myelitis. Usually it involves one segment of the cord. When the lesion extends over three or more vertebral segments, it is known as longitudinally extensive transverse myelitis (LETM) or long-segment transverse myelitis (LSTM). Dengue virus can affect any segment of the spinal cord but thoracic segments are most commonly affected [57]. The spinal cord involvement during the course of dengue infection is extremely rare [58–61]. Acute transverse myelitis [62] is a type of spinal cord involvement observed among dengue patients. Acute transverse myelitis (ATM) may occur during the course of DVI or post-infection. Post-infectious immune-mediated myelitis usually develops within 14 days after the onset of initial symptoms [61], whereas parainfectious myelitis can occur among patients within the first 7 days of infection [7, 59, 60, 63, 64].

6.6.1   Pathogenesis of Dengue-Induced Transverse Myelitis

Both viral neurotropism and post-infectious mechanisms are involved in the pathogenesis of dengue-associated myelitis. DENV is pathogenic to the neural tissues, and this direct pathogenic effect is evident by the presence viral antigen in CSF of patients. Viral antigen in the CSF can be detected during the early stage of the infection [60]. Moreover, viral antigens can be isolated from the brain, brainstem, and spinal cord where the virus can infect neural tissues. However, studies on animal models suggested the replication of DENV within the nervous system from where virus can spread to the spinal cord through CSF [65]. The pathogenesis of post-infectious myelitis revolves around the transient autoimmune reactions against myelin or other self-antigens, possibly by molecular mimicry or by nonspecific activation of auto-reactive T-cell clones [64].

6.6.2   Clinical Manifestations of Dengue-Induced Transverse Myelitis

Traverse myelitis is associated with typical symptoms including episodes of sharp pain in the lower back, legs, and arms, sensations of numbness, tickling, coldness and burning, weakness in arms and legs, and irregular bladder and bowel movements [8].

6.6.3   Diagnosis of Dengue-Induced Transverse Myelitis

Since inflammatory demyelinating lesions are manifested in transverse myelitis, the sudden onset of sensorimotor and sphincter disturbances might be observed among patients [11]. On the other hand, spinal lesions are extended to three or more vertebral segments in LETM [66]. Transverse myelitis can be broadly classified into four categories [67]:

1. Demyelination (monofocal clinical isolated syndrome) or multifocal demyelination (acute disseminated encephalomyelitis—ADEM—or multiple sclerosis)
2. Combined systemic connective tissue disease
3. Infectious
4. Idiopathic illness

Findings from spinal MRI must be positive to establish the confirmed diagnosis of TM/LETM. The diagnosis of transverse myelitis is also supported by hyperintensity in T2-weighted signals found in spinal MRI. However, inflammatory reactions in the CSF have also been observed in most of the cases. It is important to note that myelitis can also be caused by other arbovirus infections such as chikungunya, West Nile, and Zika. These infections must be ruled out during the diagnostic workup [8].

6.6.4   Management of Dengue-Induced Transverse Myelitis

The administration of intravenous (IV) steroids shows satisfactory recovery among patients, particularly those with parainfectious transverse myelitis [68]. The prime objective of treatment for transverse myelitis includes alleviation of symptoms and reduction of spinal cord inflammation. The cause of transverse myelitis needs to be addressed. Initial treatment includes intravenous corticosteroids which not only reduce swelling and inflammation in the spine but also reduce activity of immune system. Usually methylprednisolone or dexamethasone is administered intravenously for a period of 5–7 days. Intravenous corticosteroids also help in reducing subsequent attacks of transverse myelitis. People who don't respond well to intravenous steroids are treated with plasmapheresis. Intravenous immunoglobulin (IVIG) is another modality of treatment which is thought to stabilize the deranged immune system. Antiviral medications may help among patients with other suspected viral causes myelitis. Aggressive physiotherapy should be considered for all patients. In most of the cases of transverse myelitis, the process of recovery is time taking which usually takes around 3 months following the attack. Recovery may continue for up to 2 years and even longer in few cases. However, it is suggested that if there is no improvement in the patient's conditions within the first 6 months of injury, complete recovery is unlikely. Prompt and aggressive treatment with corticosteroids, IVIG, and physiotherapy has been shown to improve the prognosis [11].

6.7   Dengue-Induced Acute Disseminated Encephalomyelitis (ADEM)

Acute disseminated encephalomyelitis (ADEM) may occur during or after the DVI. It is characterized by an acute inflammatory demyelinating ailment affecting the CNS. As a monophasic course, it is also associated with multifocal white matter involvement [56]. The prevalence of ADEM in dengue infection is very low, and there are only few cases in isolated case reports [8]. Patients may present with ADEM after 5–6 days of onset of initial signs and symptoms [69].

6.7.1   Pathogenesis of Dengue-Induced ADEM

Immune reactions are primarily involved in the pathogenesis of dengue-related ADEM [69]. These reactions are autoimmune in nature which occur against myelin or to unknown self-antigens [64].

6.7.2   Clinical Manifestations of Dengue-Induced ADEM

Patients with dengue-induced ADEM present with typical sensory and motor symptoms which may develop after 1–2 weeks of infection. The following neurological manifestations may occur among dengue patients with ADEM [70, 71]:

- Disturbance in consciousness
- Disturbances in language/speaking
- Paresis
- Sensorial deficits
- Altered sensorium

6.7.3   Diagnosis of Dengue-Induced ADEM

CSF examination may assist in the diagnosis of ADEM. However, it is important to note that normal CSF cannot disregard the possibility of ADEM [72]. CSF examination may show mild pleocytosis and moderate increase in protein concentration [35]. Findings from MRIs show extensive involvement of the white matter of the frontal, parietal, or temporal lobe, basal ganglia, brainstem, cerebellum, corpus callosum, and periventricular lesions [23, 56, 69, 73]. Histological examination of lesions can show macrophage influx, perivenous demyelination, and perivascular infiltration of lymphocytes with hemorrhagic foci [74, 75]. Moreover, abnormalities in the spinal cord may be observed primarily in the thoracic and cervical regions [35].

6.7.4   Management of Dengue-Induced ADEM

There is no specific or established treatment for ADEM. Several studies have demonstrated promising role of corticosteroids during active phase [64, 69, 73]. Dengue patients with ADEM portend favorable outcome. However, persistent neurological symptoms have been observed in some patients. Early diagnosis is critical for a good prognosis [70, 74, 75].

6.8   Neuromyelitis Optica (NMO) and Optical Neuritis (ON)

Neuromyelitis optica (NMO) or Devic's syndrome is an autoimmune and inflammatory disorder involving both optic nerve and spinal cord which results in decreased visual acuity and spinal cord disorder. The optic nerve and spinal cord are involved either simultaneously or separately resulting in symmetrical weakness, reduced sensation, and loss of control on bladder and bowel movements. Both NMO and isolated optical neuritis (ON) have been reported in isolated cases in association with previous DVI [76–78].

6.8.1   Pathogenesis of Dengue-Induced NMO and ON

The pathogenesis of dengue-induced NMO and ON is poorly understood. Since NMO is a type of ADEM, similar pathological mechanisms can be applied [79].

6.8.2   Clinical Manifestations of Dengue-Induced NMO and ON

Dengue-associated ON is primarily characterized by the acute loss of vision. Fundoscopic evaluation may show papilla edema among patients [78]. On the other hand, dengue-associated NMO is primarily associated with acute loss of vision, weakness of the lower limbs, hyperreflexia, and Babinski sign [79].

6.8.3   Diagnosis of Dengue-Induced NMO and ON

NMO and ON can be identified with clinical signs along with MR imaging. MR imaging may present normal results for the brain and show a hypointensive lesion of the spinal cord. Ophthalmological examination reveals bilateral involvement of the optic nerve, with severe visual impairment in one or both eyes and bilateral papilla edema. Serial computed campimetry can be used to evaluate the recovery [79].

6.8.4 Treatment of Dengue-Induced NMO and ON

Treatment may include pulse therapy with intravenous (IV) methylprednisolone followed by oral prednisone in decreasing doses [79].

6.9 Dengue-Induced Guillain–Barré Syndrome

Guillain–Barré syndrome (GBS) features a quickly rising paralysis, reflecting an inflammatory demyelinating or axonal polyneuropathy. GBS following dengue virus infection is uncommon and has been described in few case reports primarily in children than adults [8]. It has been reported that GBS accounts for 30% of the neurological manifestations of DVI [32]. GBS has also been described in patients with oligosymptomatic dengue virus infection [80]. Moreover, dengue-associated Miller Fisher syndrome has been reported in the literature [81].

6.9.1 Pathogenesis of Dengue-Induced Guillain–Barré Syndrome

Cell-mediated immunological reactions are primarily involved in the pathogenesis of GBS. Activated T cells could cross the vascular endothelium (blood–brain barrier) and recognize an antigen in the endoneural compartment. Both cytokines and chemokines are produced by T cells which cause the opening of the blood–brain barrier resulting in the entry of antibodies and Schwann cells to attack. These immunological events are triggered by dengue virus, leading to the GBS. Myelin or axons could be the target of this immune response [23].

6.9.2 Clinical Manifestations of Dengue-Induced Guillain–Barré Syndrome

GBS is clinically manifested by acute onset of weakness in the limbs. Moreover, it is also associated with areflexia. Electrophysiological studies may demonstrate the demyelination of peripheral nerves which indicate the motor and sensory nerves' involvement. The neurological spectrum of GBS during the course of DVI corresponds to GBS resulting from other infectious diseases. In both cases, ascending paraparesis is the primary manifestation of GBS [80]. Fever, pain, exanthema, arthralgia, decrease in muscle power and tone, and involvement of respiratory and facial muscles are primary clinical presentations of GBS in dengue [82].

6.9.3   Diagnosis of Dengue-Induced Guillain–Barré Syndrome

Dengue-induced GBS can be diagnosed with clinical findings along with CSF examination. CSF analysis might show increased protein concentrations without pleocytosis (albumin-cytological dissociation) [73].

6.9.4   Management of Dengue-Induced Guillain–Barré Syndrome

Dengue-induced GBS can be managed with supportive treatments. However, plasma exchange is also a mainstay of therapy. Findings from randomized trials suggest plasma exchange be more effective than supportive care during the management of GBS. Moreover, intravenous administration of immunoglobulins has demonstrated similar effectiveness as of plasma exchange and might be more advantageous. Limited data on the efficacy of corticosteroids alone do not support its use in the treatment of GBS. CSF filtration is another treatment option, but it requires more clinical investigations to establish its use for GBS [8, 83]. Dengue-induced GBS demonstrate good prognosis with timely and appropriate measures [82].

6.10   Dengue-Induced Hypokalemic Paralysis

Hypokalemic paralysis is clinically manifested as flaccid generalized weakness which is caused by the reduction of serum potassium levels. It can occur either spontaneously or due to some triggers. Insulin or glucose administration plays a pivotal role in triggering the hypokalemic paralysis. Mutations in both sodium and potassium channels contributed hypokalemic periodic paralysis. On the basis of these mutations, hypokalemic paralysis is characterized into two types including [84]:

1. Type 1 hypokalemic paralysis (due to mutation in CACNL1A3 calcium channel gene)
2. Type 2 hypokalemic paralysis (due to mutation SCN4A sodium channel gene)

There are several other conditions during which periodic paralysis associated with low serum potassium may be observed. These conditions include thyrotoxicosis, primary hyperaldosteronism, and Sjogren syndrome with distal renal tubular acidosis [62, 85]. Recently, dengue has been reported as a cause of hypokalemic paralysis in individual cases and small case series [8]. Dengue myositis and idiopathic hypokalemic paralysis are closely related to hypokalemic paralysis. However, these conditions vary from each other in terms of clinical characteristics, biochemical features, and consequences [13].

6.10.1 Pathogenesis of Dengue-Induced Hypokalemic Paralysis

The pathogenesis of hypokalemic paralysis in dengue remains obscure. It can be hypothesized that hypokalemia during the course of DVI might be attributed to serum potassium redistribution in cells and increased urinary excretion of potassium due to transient renal tubular dysfunction. The occurrence of hypokalemic acute kidney injury has recently emerged among dengue patient. These findings support the hypothesis of hypokalemic paralysis in DVI [13, 86–88]. Furthermore, infection-related stress plays a pivotal role in the pathogenesis of hypokalemia. Infectious stress may cause the release of catecholamine or insulin, which results in an intracellular shift of potassium [87, 89].

The leakage of plasma through vascular wall is considered to be central in the pathogenesis of dengue-induced hypokalemia. Unlike other hemorrhagic viral infections, overt endothelial damage and cytopathic effects on endothelial cells are not indicated in DVI [90, 91]. The endothelial damage during the course of DVI might be triggered by antibodies secreted by B lymphocytes and cytokines involved in the cell-mediated immunity. These cytokines include tumor necrosis factor alpha (TNF-α), interferon-gamma (IFN-γ), and interleukins (IL-2, IL-6, IL-1β, and IL-8) [91]. Activation of endothelial cells enhances this inflammatory response, resulting in overexpression of various chemokines and vascular endothelial growth factor (VEGF) [90]. The endothelial dysfunction results in loss of fluid and electrolytes out of vascular compartment and reduction in serum potassium levels. Moreover, kidney function impairment caused by glomerular, tubular, interstitial, or vascular endothelial damage is another important factor associated with hypokalemia in DVI [85]. Dengue-induced acute kidney injury with hypokalemia is a highly morbid and fatal complication of DVI [88].

6.10.2 Clinical Manifestations of Dengue-Induced Hypokalemic Paralysis

Hypokalemic paralysis in dengue is presented with generalized weakness in all four limbs. Neck, facial, and bulbar weakness has been observed in several patients [85].

6.10.3 Diagnosis of Dengue-Induced Hypokalemic Paralysis

Hypokalemic paralysis caused by dengue should be differentiated from periodic paralysis caused by urinary potassium wasting syndromes, alcohol abuse, and myasthenia gravis. Low levels of serum potassium and elevated creatine kinase levels are associated with hypokalemic paralytic episodes. The elevated levels of creatine phosphokinase result from vasoconstriction and muscular ischemia due to hypokalemia [92]. The severity of muscle weakness is always correlated with potassium levels [13]. Hypokalemia without paralysis has been observed in several patients [93]. Hypomagnesemia is also documented in relation with paralysis along with hypokalemia [86].

6.10.4 Management of Dengue-Induced Hypokalemic Paralysis

Dengue-associated hypokalemic paralysis can be effectively managed with potassium supplementation. Studies have shown satisfactory recovery of dengue patients with hypokalemic paralysis following the intravenous administration of potassium [87]. Hypokalemic paralysis can occur along with hypomagnesemia. It has been observed that weakness may persist even after potassium supplementation, in the presence of low serum magnesium levels. However, complete recovery can be observed within 48–72 h, with a normalization of serum potassium and magnesium levels. This mechanism can be explained by the relationship between potassium and magnesium. Hypomagnesemia inhibits muscle Na+ and K+-ATPase activity resulting in reduced ion influx into the muscle fibers and secondary kaliuresis [86].

6.11   Dengue-Induced Neuritis

The prevalence of dengue-induced neuritis is quite low. Neuritis during the course of DVI is reported by individual case reports. Neuritis has varying manifestations among dengue patients ranging from brachial neuritis, long thoracic/phrenic/abducens nerve palsy, and peripheral facial palsy [8].

6.11.1 Pathogenesis of Dengue-Induced Neuritis

The exact mechanism underlying the pathogenesis of DVI-related neuritis is unclear. However, evidence of immune reactions has been well established in the literature [7].

6.11.2 Clinical Manifestations of Dengue-Induced Neuritis

The clinical manifestations of neuritis in dengue infection are primarily dependent on the location of lesions. Patients may experience neuropathic pain or weakness and atrophy of the proximal musculature, mainly of the upper limbs. These manifestations are attributed to the involvement of the brachial plexus [19].

6.11.3 Diagnosis of Dengue-Induced Neuritis

Diagnosis of dengue-induced neuritis is well established. The first and foremost diagnostic consideration is to exclude other causes of neuritis. These may include infections, tumor, traumas, demyelinating diseases, and stroke. Neurophysiological examination includes motor or sensory evaluation of nerves. These evaluations should be extended to axillary, musculocutaneous, suprascapular, long thoracic, radial, median, and ulnar nerves. The findings originated from these evaluations may reveal reduced amplitudes suggesting axonal degeneration. Electromyography evaluation should be carried out for suspected patients [19].

6.11.4 Management of Dengue-Induced Neuritis

Dengue-associated nerve palsy can be managed with supportive care, steroids, and intravenous immunoglobulins. Most of the cases demonstrate satisfactory recovery with supportive treatment. Corticosteroids or intravenous immunoglobulins are not required by all patients and some may improve without any specific treatment [14, 94]. However, many cases respond well with administration of steroids only [19].

6.12   Diagnostic Considerations of Dengue-Induced Neurological Complications

Dengue-induced neurological complications can be identified through dengue IgM, viral antigens, or RNA. However, diagnosis becomes difficult due to the possibility of neurological involvement in oligosymptomatic or asymptomatic dengue cases. Hematological tests, CSF analysis, and MRI findings are of paramount importance in such cases. These tests not only assist in the diagnosis neurological complications but also aid to exclude other factors contributing neurological symptoms. All the suspected cases must be referred for the following diagnostic workup [23]:

- Blood tests
- Biochemical profile
- Hepatic function tests
- Test for rheumatic diseases
- Tests for hepatitis B and C
- Test for human immunodeficiency virus-1 (HIV-1)
- CSF analysis
  - Cell count (total or specific).
  - Quantification of protein concentration in CSF.
  - Quantification of glucose and lactate concentration in CSF.
  - Identification of bacteria and fungi through smear and culture techniques.
  - Evaluation of normality and functioning of blood–CSF barrier by using albumin quotient (CSF/serum).
  - Identification of intrathecal production of total immunoglobulin G.
  - Quantification of specific antibodies against other pathogens in order to assist differential diagnosis. These pathogens may include *Treponema pallidum* (syphilis), herpes simplex virus, Epstein–Barr virus, and cytomegalovirus.

The results of CSF examination can be normal, but it does not exclude the possibility of neurological intricacies. Dengue encephalitis may appear with normal CSF in up to 50% of cases [32]. Nevertheless, the importance of CSF analysis should be disregarded during the diagnosis of neurological complications in DVI. Dengue-specific antibodies (IgM and IgG), RNA, or viral antigen should also be evaluated for suspected cases [95]. The specificity of ELISA for detection of dengue IgM is very high (97–100%). However, this technique has wide disparity in sensitivity which may range from 0 to 73%, depending on the method used. It might be possible that CSF analysis shows absence of specific IgM but these results do not exclude the plausibility of dengue infection as a precursor of neurological diseases [32, 95, 96]. Caution must be carried out during the diagnostic workup as IgG may present in CSF due to prior infection and has tendency to cross blood–CSF barrier. In this context, relying only on presence of IgG in CSF may overestimate the neurological complications in dengue infection [23]. On the other hand, NS1 antigen can be detected in CSF by using ELISA with sensitivity of 50% and specificity of 100%. However, combined identification of NS1 Ag and specific IgM in CSF increases the sensitivity of diagnosis up to 92% [95].

PCR identification of viral RNA in CSF is also a useful tool, but it may produce varying results ranging from 0 to 83%. Such wide discrepancies might be attributed to the different viral phenotypes which have distinct neurovirulent and neuroinvasive properties. Other factor that may contribute to such variations is disease stage, as viral RNA can only be detected during acute phase of disease. It must be considered that not all dengue-related neurological complications are due to direct virus neuroinvasion and some cases do not have RNA in CSF. However, the absence of viral RNA in CSF does not exclude the diagnosis of neurological manifestation due to dengue infection [27, 95, 96].

Another consideration during the diagnosis of DENV-associated neurological complications includes understandings of pattern and transmission cycle of virus. High virus circulation and transmission, particularly in dengue-hyperendemic regions, increase the probability of secondary infection and hence of severe clinical manifestations including nervous system involvements. Such pattern is primarily observed in the regions with distinct serotype circulation. In order to understand the exact disease pathogenesis, reliability of diagnostic method is of utmost importance. There is a dire need to develop and validate new diagnostic tools. The applications of nucleic acid tests (NATs) in CSF would be of paramount importance in this regard [56].

References

1. Horstick O, Jaenisch T, Martinez E, Kroeger A, See LLC, Farrar J, et al. Comparing the usefulness of the 1997 and 2009 WHO dengue case classification: a systematic literature review. Am J Trop Med Hyg. 2014;91(3):621–34.
2. World Health Organization, Special Programme for Research and Training in Tropical Diseases, World Health Organization. Department of Control of Neglected Tropical Diseases,

World Health Organization. Epidemic and Pandemic Alert and Response. Dengue: guidelines for diagnosis, treatment, prevention and control. Geneva: World Health Organization; 2009.

3. Nimmannitya S, Thisyakorn U, Hemsrichart V. Dengue haemorrhagic fever with unusual manifestations. Southeast Asian J Trop Med Public Health. 1987;18(3):398–406.

4. Kho L, Wulur H, Jahja E, Gubler D. Dengue hemorrhagic fever accompanied by encephalopathy in Jakarta. Southeast Asian J Trop Med Public Health. 1981;12(1):83–6.

5. Hendarto S, Hadinegoro R. Dengue encephalopathy. Pediatr Int. 1992;34(3):350–7.

6. Sanguansermsri T, Poneprasert B, Phornphutkul B, Kulapongs P, Tantachamrun T. Acute encephalopathy associated with dengue infection. Bangkok: Seameo Tropmed; 1976. p. 10–1.

7. Carod-Artal FJ, Wichmann O, Farrar J, Gascón J. Neurological complications of dengue virus infection. Lancet Neurol. 2013;12(9):906–19.

8. Li G-H, Ning Z-J, Liu Y-M, Li X-H. Neurological manifestations of dengue infection. Front Cell Infect Microbiol. 2017;7:449.

9. Varatharaj A. Encephalitis in the clinical spectrum of dengue infection. Neurol India. 2010;58(4):585.

10. Bhat RY, Varma C. Meningitis as a primary presentation of dengue infection. J Microbiol Infect Dis. 2013;3(01):39–40.

11. Scott T, Frohman E, De Seze J, Gronseth G, Weinshenker BG. Evidence-based guideline: clinical evaluation and treatment of transverse myelitis: report of the Therapeutics and Technology Assessment Subcommittee of the American Academy of Neurology. Neurology. 2011;77(24):2128–34.

12. Solbrig MV, Perng G-C. Current neurological observations and complications of dengue virus infection. Curr Neurol Neurosci Rep. 2015;15(6):29.

13. Maurya PK, Kulshreshtha D, Singh AK, Thacker AK. Rapidly resolving weakness related to hypokalemia in patients infected with dengue virus. J Clin Neuromuscul Dis. 2016;18(2):72–8.

14. Peter S, Malhotra N, Peter P, Sood R. Isolated Bell's palsy—an unusual presentation of dengue infection. Asian Pac J Trop Med. 2013;6(1):82–4.

15. Cam B, Fonsmark L, Hue N, Phuong N, Poulsen A, Heegaard E. Prospective case-control study of encephalopathy in children with dengue hemorrhagic fever. Am J Trop Med Hyg. 2001;65(6):848–51.

16. Pancharoen C, Thisyakorn U. Neurological manifestations in dengue patients. Southeast Asian J Trop Med Public Health. 2001;32(2):341–5.

17. Solomon T, Dung NM, Vaughn DW, Kneen R, Raengsakulrach B, Loan HT, et al. Neurological manifestations of dengue infection. Lancet. 2000;355(9209):1053–9.

18. Sharma CM, Kumawat B, Ralot T, Tripathi G, Dixit S. Guillain-Barre syndrome occurring during dengue fever. J Indian Med Assoc. 2011;109(9):675, 682.

19. Verma R, Sharma P, Khurana N, Sharma L. Neuralgic amyotrophy associated with dengue fever: case series of three patients. J Postgrad Med. 2011;57(4):329.

20. Lum L, Lam SK, Choy Y, George R, Harun F. Dengue encephalitis: a true entity? Am J Trop Med Hyg. 1996;54(3):256–9.

21. Thisyakorn U, Thisyakorn C, Limpitikul W, Nisalak A. Dengue infection with central nervous system manifestations. Southeast Asian J Trop Med Public Health. 1999;30(3):504–6.

22. Chaturvedi U, Dhawan R, Khanna M, Mathur A. Breakdown of the blood-brain barrier during dengue virus infection of mice. J Gen Virol. 1991;72(4):859–66.

23. Puccioni-Sohler M, Orsini M, Soares CN. Dengue: a new challenge for neurology. Neurol Int. 2012;4(3):e15.

24. Ramos C, SÁNchez G, Pando RH, Baquera J, Hernández D, Mota J, et al. Dengue virus in the brain of a fatal case of hemorrhagic dengue fever: case report. J Neurovirol. 1998;4(4):465–8.

25. Salazar MI, Richardson JH, Sánchez-Vargas I, Olson KE, Beaty BJ. Dengue virus type 2: replication and tropisms in orally infected Aedes aegypti mosquitoes. BMC Microbiol. 2007;7(1):9.

26. Lima DM, de Paula SO, de Oliveira Franca RF, Palma PV, Morais FR, Gomes-Ruiz AC, et al. A DNA vaccine candidate encoding the structural prM/E proteins elicits a strong immune response and protects mice against dengue-4 virus infection. Vaccine. 2011;29(4):831–8.

27. Domingues RB, Kuster GW, Onuki-Castro FL, Souza VA, Levi JE, Pannuti CS. Involvement of the central nervous system in patients with dengue virus infection. J Neurol Sci. 2008;267(1-2):36–40.
28. Soares C, Cabral-Castro M, Peralta J, Freitas M, Puccioni-Sohler M. Meningitis determined by oligosymptomatic dengue virus type 3 infection: report of a case. Int J Infect Dis. 2010;14(2):e150–e2.
29. Miagostovich MP, dos Santos FB, Fumian TM, Guimarães FR, da Costa EV, Tavares FN, et al. Complete genetic characterization of a Brazilian dengue virus type 3 strain isolated from a fatal outcome. Mem Inst Oswaldo Cruz. 2006;101(3):307–13.
30. Schmitz J, Roehrig J, Barrett A, Hombach J. Next generation dengue vaccines: a review of candidates in preclinical development. Vaccine. 2011;29(42):7276–84.
31. Simmons CP, Farrar J. Changing patterns of dengue epidemiology and implications for clinical management and vaccines. PLoS Med. 2009;6(9):e1000129.
32. Soares C, Faria L, Peralta J, De Freitas M, Puccioni-Sohler M. Dengue infection: neurological manifestations and cerebrospinal fluid (CSF) analysis. J Neurol Sci. 2006;249(1):19–24.
33. Misra U, Kalita J, Syam U, Dhole T. Neurological manifestations of dengue virus infection. J Neurol Sci. 2006;244(1–2):117–22.
34. Jackson S, Mullings A, Bennett F, Khan C, Gordon-Strachan G, Rhoden T. Dengue infection in patients presenting with neurological manifestations in a dengue endemic population. West Indian Med J. 2008;57(4):373–6.
35. Wasay M, Channa R, Jumani M, Shabbir G, Azeemuddin M, Zafar A. Encephalitis and myelitis associated with dengue viral infection: clinical and neuroimaging features. Clin Neurol Neurosurg. 2008;110(6):635–40.
36. Innis B, Myint K, Nisalak A, Ishak K, Nimmannitya S, Laohapand T, et al. Acute liver failure is one important cause of fatal dengue infection. Southeast Asian J Trop Med Public Health. 1990;21:695–6.
37. Angibaud G, Luaute J, Laille M, Gaultier C. Brain involvement in dengue fever. J Clin Neurosci. 2001;8(1):63–5.
38. Gupta VK, Lalchandani A, Agrawal K. Neurological manifestations of dengue infection. Ann Trop Med Public Health. 2015;8(4):117.
39. Hommel D, Talarmin A, Deubel V, Reynes J, Drouet M, Sarthou J, et al. Dengue encephalitis in French Guiana. Res Virol. 1998;149(4):235–8.
40. Baldaçara L, Ferreira JR, Filho LCPS, Venturini RR, Coutinho OMVC, Camargo WC, et al. Behavior disorder after encephalitis caused by dengue. J Neuropsychiatr Clin Neurosci. 2013;25(1):E44.
41. Verma R, Sharma P, Garg RK, Atam V, Singh MK, Mehrotra HS. Neurological complications of dengue fever: experience from a tertiary center of north India. Ann Indian Acad Neurol. 2011;14(4):272.
42. Malavige G, Ranatunga P, Jayaratne S, Wijesiriwardana B, Seneviratne S, Karunatilaka D. Dengue viral infections as a cause of encephalopathy. Indian J Med Microbiol. 2007;25(2):143.
43. Soares CN, Cabral-Castro MJ, Peralta JM, de Freitas MR, Zalis M, Puccioni-Sohler M. Review of the etiologies of viral meningitis and encephalitis in a dengue endemic region. J Neurol Sci. 2011;303(1-2):75–9.
44. Bordignon J, Strottmann DM, Mosimann ALP, Probst CM, Stella V, Noronha L, et al. Dengue neurovirulence in mice: identification of molecular signatures in the E and NS3 helicase domains. J Med Virol. 2007;79(10):1506–17.
45. Verma R, Varatharaj A. Epilepsia partialis continua as a manifestation of dengue encephalitis. Epilepsy Behav. 2011;20(2):395–7.
46. Soares C, Puccioni-Sohler M. Dengue encephalitis: suggestion for case definition. J Neurol Sci. 2011;306(1):165.
47. Kennedy P. Viral encephalitis: causes, differential diagnosis, and management. J Neurol Neurosurg Psychiatry. 2004;75(suppl 1):i10–i5.

48. Muzaffar J, Venkata PK, Gupta N, Kar P. Dengue encephalitis: why we need to identify this entity in a dengue-prone region. Singap Med J. 2006;47(11):975–7.
49. Borawake K, Prayag P, Wagh A, Dole S. Dengue encephalitis. Indian J Crit Care Med. 2011;15(3):190.
50. Baheti G, Mehta V, Ramchandani M, Ghosh GC. Dengue fever with encephalitis: a rare phenomenon. BMJ Case Rep. 2018;2018:bcr-2018-225463.
51. Weeratunga PN, Caldera MC, Gooneratne IK, Gamage R, Perera P. Neurological manifestations of dengue: a cross sectional study. Travel Med Infect Dis. 2014;12(2):189–93.
52. Qui PT, Hue NB, Bao LQ, Van Cam B, Khanh TH, Hien TT, et al. Viral etiology of encephalitis in children in southern Vietnam: results of a one-year prospective descriptive study. PLoS Negl Trop Dis. 2010;4(10):e854.
53. Kumar S, Prabhakar S. Guillain-Barre syndrome occurring in the course of dengue fever. Neurol India. 2005;53(2):250–1.
54. Goswami RP, Mukherjee A, Biswas T, Karmakar PS, Ghosh A. Two cases of dengue meningitis: a rare first presentation. J Infect Dev Ctries. 2012;6(02):208–11.
55. Mamdouh KH, Mroog KM, Hani NH, Nabil EM. Atypical dengue meningitis in makkah, saudi arabia with slow resolving, prominent migraine like headache, phobia, and arrhythmia. J Global Infect Dis. 2013;5(4):183.
56. Puccioni-Sohler M, Rosadas C, Cabral-Castro MJ. Neurological complications in dengue infection: a review for clinical practice. Arq Neuropsiquiatr. 2013;71(9B):667–71.
57. Nandasiri S, Wimalaratna H, Manjula M, Corea E. Transverse myelitis secondary to melioidosis; a case report. BMC Infect Dis. 2012;12(1):232.
58. Renganathan A, Ng WK, Tan CT. Transverse myelitis in association with dengue infection. Neurol J Southeast Asia. 1996;1(1):61–3.
59. Leão RN, Oikawa T, Rosa ES, Yamaki JT, Rodrigues SG, Vasconcelos HB, et al. Isolation of dengue 2 virus from a patient with central nervous system involvement (transverse myelitis). Rev Soc Bras Med Trop. 2002;35(4):401–4.
60. Kunishige M, Mitsui T, Tan B, Leong H, Takasaki T, Kurane I, et al. Preferential gray matter involvement in dengue myelitis. Neurology. 2004;63(10):1980–1.
61. Seet RC, Lim EC, Wilder-Smith EP. Acute transverse myelitis following dengue virus infection. J Clin Virol. 2006;35(3):310–2.
62. Alkaabi JM, Mushtaq A, Al-Maskari FN, Moussa NA, Gariballa S. Hypokalemic periodic paralysis: a case series, review of the literature and update of management. Eur J Emerg Med. 2010;17(1):45–7.
63. Landais A, Hartz B, Alhendi R, Lannuzel A. Acute myelitis associated with dengue infection. Med Mal Infect. 2018;49(4):270–4.
64. Murthy J. Neurological complications of dengue infection. Neurol India. 2010;58(4):581.
65. An J, Zhou D-S, Kawasaki K, Yasui K. The pathogenesis of spinal cord involvement in dengue virus infection. Virchows Arch. 2003;442(5):472–81.
66. Wolf VL, Lupo PJ, Lotze TE. Pediatric acute transverse myelitis overview and differential diagnosis. J Child Neurol. 2012;27(11):1426–36.
67. Jacob A, Weinshenker BG, editors. An approach to the diagnosis of acute transverse myelitis. Semin Neurol. 2008;28(1):105–20.
68. Fong CY, Hlaing CS, Tay CG, Kadir KAA, Goh KJ, Ong LC. Longitudinal extensive transverse myelitis with cervical epidural haematoma following dengue virus infection. Eur J Paediatr Neurol. 2016;20(3):449–53.
69. Gupta M, Nayak R, Khwaja GA, Chowdhury D. Acute disseminated encephalomyelitis associated with dengue infection: a case report with literature review. J Neurol Sci. 2013;335(1–2):216–8.
70. Gera C, George U. Acute disseminating encephalomyelitis with hemorrhage following dengue. Neurol India. 2010;58(4):595.
71. Brito CA, Sobreira S, Cordeiro MT, Lucena-Silva N. Acute disseminated encephalomyelitis in classic dengue. Rev Soc Bras Med Trop. 2007;40(2):236–8.

72. Viswanathan S, Botross N, Rusli B, Riad A. Acute disseminated encephalomyelitis complicating dengue infection with neuroimaging mimicking multiple sclerosis: a report of two cases. Mult Scler Relat Disord. 2016;10:112–5.
73. Domingues R, Kuster G. Diagnosis and management neurologic manifestations associated with acute dengue virus infection. J Neuroinfect Dis. 2014;5(138):2.
74. Yamamoto Y, Hitani A, Nakamura T, Iwamoto A, Takasaki T, Yamada K-I, et al. Acute disseminated encephalomyelitis following dengue fever. J Infect Chemother. 2002;8(2):175–7.
75. Sundaram C, Uppin SG, Dakshinamurthy K, Borgahain R. Acute disseminated encephalomyelitis following dengue hemorrhagic fever. Neurol India. 2010;58(4):599.
76. Pittock SJ, Weinshenker BG, Lucchinetti CF, Wingerchuk DM, Corboy JR, Lennon VA. Neuromyelitis optica brain lesions localized at sites of high aquaporin 4 expression. Arch Neurol. 2006;63(7):964–8.
77. Preechawat P, Poonyathalang A. Bilateral optic neuritis after dengue viral infection. J Neuroophthalmol. 2005;25(1):51–2.
78. de Aragão REM, Barreira IMA, Lima LNC, Rabelo LP, Pereira FBA. Bilateral optic neuritis after dengue viral infection: case report. Arq Bras Oftalmol. 2010;73(2):175–8.
79. de Sousa AM, Puccioni-Sohler M, Alvarenga MP, Alvarenga RMP, Borges AD, Adorno LF. Post-dengue neuromyelitis optica: case report of a Japanese-descendent Brazilian child. J Infect Chemother. 2006;12(6):396–8.
80. Bhoopat L, Bhamarapravati N, Attasiri C, Yoksarn S, Chaiwun B, Khunamornpong S, et al. Immunohistochemical characterization of a new monoclonal antibody reactive with dengue virus-infected cells in frozen tissue using immunoperoxidase technique. Asian Pac J Allergy Immunol. 1996;14(2):107.
81. Gaultier C, Angibaud G, Laille M, Lacassin F. Probable syndrome de Miller Fisher au cours d'une dengue de type 2. Rev Neurol. 2000;156(2):169–71.
82. Keesen TSL, de Almeida RP, Gois BM, Peixoto RF, Pachá ASC, Vieira FCF, et al. Guillain-Barré syndrome and arboviral infection in Brazil. Lancet Infect Dis. 2017;17(7):693–4.
83. Qureshi N, Begum A, Saha P, Hossain M. Guillain-Barre syndrome following dengue fever in adult patient. J Med. 2012;13(2):246–9.
84. Miller T, Da Silva MD, Miller H, Kwiecinski H, Mendell J, Tawil R, et al. Correlating phenotype and genotype in the periodic paralyses. Neurology. 2004;63(9):1647–55.
85. Verma R, Patil TB, Lalla R. Hypokalemic paralysis associated with dengue fever: study from a tertiary centre in North India. Neurol Asia. 2016;21:1.
86. Jain RS, Gupta PK, Agrawal R, Kumar S, Khandelwal K. An unusual case of dengue infection presenting with hypokalemic paralysis with hypomagnesemia. J Clin Virol. 2015;69:197–9.
87. Jha S, Ansari M. Dengue infection causing acute hypokalemic quadriparesis. Neurol India. 2010;58(4):592.
88. Mallhi TH, Khan AH, Adnan AS, Sarriff A, Khan YH, Jummaat F. Incidence, characteristics and risk factors of acute kidney injury among dengue patients: a retrospective analysis. PLoS One. 2015;10:9.
89. Hira HS, Kaur A, Shukla A. Acute neuromuscular weakness associated with dengue infection. J Neurosci Rural Pract. 2012;3(1):36.
90. Spiropoulou CF, Srikiatkhachorn A. The role of endothelial activation in dengue hemorrhagic fever and hantavirus pulmonary syndrome. Virulence. 2013;4(6):525–36.
91. Martina BE, Koraka P, Osterhaus AD. Dengue virus pathogenesis: an integrated view. Clin Microbiol Rev. 2009;22(4):564–81.
92. Paliwal VK, Garg RK, Juyal R, Husain N, Verma R, Sharma PK, et al. Acute dengue virus myositis: a report of seven patients of varying clinical severity including two cases with severe fulminant myositis. J Neurol Sci. 2011;300(1–2):14–8.
93. Ying R, Tang X, Zhang F, Cai W, Chen Y, Wang J, et al. Clinical characteristics of the patients with dengue fever seen from 2002 to 2006 in Guangzhou. Zhonghua Shi Yan He Lin Chuang Bing Du Xue Za Zhi = Zhonghua shiyan he linchuang bingduxue zazhi = Chin J Exp Clin Virol. 2007;21(2):123–5.

94. Biswas NM, Pal S. Oculomotor nerve palsy in dengue encephalitis-a rare presentation. Indian J Med Res. 2014;140(6):793.
95. Araújo F, Brilhante R, Cavalcanti L, Rocha M, Cordeiro R, Perdigão A, et al. Detection of the dengue non-structural 1 antigen in cerebral spinal fluid samples using a commercially available enzyme-linked immunosorbent assay. J Virol Methods. 2011;177(1):128–31.
96. Pancharoen C, Kulwichit W, Tantawichien T, Thisyakorn U, Thisyakorn C. Dengue infection: a global concern. J Med Assoc Thai (Chotmaihet Thangphaet). 2002;85:S25–33.

Dengue-Induced Musculoskeletal Complications

7

7.1   Musculoskeletal Involvements in Dengue Infection

Dengue viral infection (DVI) has been typically designated as "bone break fever" owing to its clinical manifestations of severe muscle soreness, joint ache, as well as bone pain. Muscle involvements in patients with DVI can be apparent in the form of myalgias, myositis, rhabdomyolysis, and hypokalemic paralysis [1]. Direct invasion of dengue virus (DENV) into the muscles has been debated since decade. However, an in vitro investigation reveals the tendency of DENV to infect and modify the calcium storage of skeletal muscle cells. This observation supports the hypothesis that skeletal muscle dysfunction during the course of DVI is a result of uninterrupted/direct infection of skeletal muscle fibers by DENV. Moreover, this study also elaborates the high susceptibility of cultured myotubes towards virus. These findings underscore that skeletal muscles are direct target organ of DENV infection. Since skeletal muscles are comprised of large tissue volume in the human body, it can be postulated that systemic increase of proinflammatory cytokines during the course of dengue infection might be attributed to the direct viral injury of the muscles [2]. However, dengue-induced musculoskeletal complications are also considered more likely to be associated with myotoxic cytokines, particularly tumor necrosis factor (TNF) [3]. Moreover, existing data elaborates that these complications can be due to a range of findings from mild lymphocytic infiltrate to foci of severe myonecrosis [3]. Muscular complications can easily be prevented with timely recognition. Urinalysis is suggested in all patients with severe dengue as a screening tool. If urinalysis is positive for heme, then serum creatinine phosphokinase (CK) levels should be measured. CK determination is the most specific test for muscular dystrophy [4], and its elevated levels are indicative of muscle disease. Since the concentration of CK is not significant in red blood cells, its levels are not affected by hemolysis. Moreover, in contrast to other functional enzymes, CK is not affected by liver dysfunctions [4]. Dengue patients may present to the hospital with pure motor weakness. Most of these cases have elevated CK along with myositis confirmed by electromyography and muscle biopsy. Overall improvement in these

© Springer Nature Singapore Pte Ltd. 2021
T. H. Mallhi et al., *Expanded Dengue Syndrome*,
https://doi.org/10.1007/978-981-15-7337-8_7

patients is satisfactory. It must be noted that dengue and dengue-related acute pure motor quadriplegia precipitated by myositis should be ruled during the differential diagnosis of acute flaccid paralysis, particularly in dengue-endemic areas [5, 6]. DVI-induced myalgias are usually short-lived but may persist after resolution of infection. However, such myalgias are subsided with initial treatment of corticosteroids [7].

7.2   Dengue-Induced Rhabdomyolysis

Rhabdomyolysis is extensive fragmentation of skeletal muscle with seepage of myocytes and their contents into the blood circulation. These muscle contents are comprised of electrolytes, myoglobin, and other sarcoplasmic proteins. Sarcoplasmic proteins include CK, lactate dehydrogenase (LDH), alanine aminotransferase (ALT), and aspartate aminotransferase [2, 8]. Rhabdomyolysis is referred to be the most severe manifestation of muscular complication during the course of DVI. Most of the cases of dengue-induced rhabdomyolysis have been recognized by isolated case reports as large histopathological investigations for identification of dengue-induced rhabdomyolysis are still not available yet. Over the last decade, there is increasing body of evidence in the literature about the association of dengue infection and rhabdomyolysis [9].

7.2.1   Clinical Manifestations
of Dengue-Induced Rhabdomyolysis

Dengue virus injury to the muscles causes myonecrosis which is clinically presented as myalgia, limb weakness, and gross pigmenturia without hematuria [10]. There is established evidence on the association of rhabdomyolysis with the development AKI and life-threatening electrolyte imbalances. Conversely, if these complications are diagnosed early, then they can be easily prevented. Usually, patients respond well to treatment, but some patients die due to multi-organ failure. Biopsy data indicate that renal injuries have been identified in several isolated cases of affected patients [11].

7.2.2   Pathogenesis of Dengue-Induced Rhabdomyolysis

The pathophysiology of the development of rhabdomyolysis during the course of DVI is not clear. It must be noted that rhabdomyolysis has been associated with various viral infections, including influenza A and B, HIV, Epstein–Barr virus, and coxsackievirus [8]. Since DENV have some common clinical characteristics with abovementioned viruses that are known to cause severe myositis, it is therefore not surprising that DENV could also cause rhabdomyolysis. Currently available data suggest involvement of myotoxic cytokines such as interferon alpha (IFN-α) and tumor necrosis factor (TNF) which are released in response to a viral infection [12]. Biopsy findings of patients having acute viral rhabdomyolysis have shown a variety of clinical findings from a mild lymphocytic infiltrate to foci of severe myonecrosis. However, direct attack of DENV into the muscles has been inconsistently reported [12]. This cytokine-mediated damage of muscle cells leads to increase in intracellular free calcium, caused by depletion of adenosine triphosphate and/or by direct injury and disruption of the plasma membrane. Increased intracellular calcium results in a cascade of chemical reactions including activation of proteases, mitochondrial abnormalities, and excessive production of reactive oxygen species that are detrimental to muscle cells. Cellular changes ultimately result in muscle cell death [1, 13]. Moreover, existing literature also provides evidence of direct viral invasion into the muscles [2].

7.2.3 Diagnosis of Dengue-Induced Rhabdomyolysis

The diagnosis of rhabdomyolysis during DVI is based on clinical manifestations. However, myoglobinuria and an elevated CK are of paramount importance. When plasma myoglobin level exceeds 0.5–1.5 mg/dL, it starts to excrete into the urine. Urinalysis must be considered in all suspected cases, and abnormal findings must be subjected to differential diagnosis of rhabdomyolysis. In many cases levels of serum CK have been observed at least 10 times of the upper limit [1, 10].

7.2.4 Management of Dengue-Induced Rhabdomyolysis

The primary management of rhabdomyolysis in DVI focuses on reversal of myoglobinuria in order to prevent the kidney injury. AKI along with myoglobinuria is the most serious and sometimes life-threatening intricacy of both traumatic and non-traumatic rhabdomyolysis. Available evidence substantially elaborates the strong association between AKI and dengue-associated rhabdomyolysis. There is still debate on the exact mechanisms of rhabdomyolysis-associated renal impairments. However, experimental evidence suggests various pathways through which muscle damage can lead to kidney dysfunctions. These pathways include direct or ischemic tubular injury, intrarenal vasoconstriction, and tubular obstruction [8]. Myoglobin concentrates in renal tubular cells where it intermingles with the Tamm–Horsfall protein resulting in its precipitation, predominantly in the presence of acidic urine. Myoglobin does not pose nephrotoxicity in tubules unless the urine is acidic. Due to this, rational urinary alkalinization is commonly used as supportive treatment measure. The low levels of CPK have been found to be associated with lower risks of AKI. Patients with CPK values less than 15,000–20,000 U/L are found to have low risks of AKI. However, there is no predictive range of serum CPK beyond which the risk of AKI substantially increases. It must be noted that AKI has been reported among patients with CPK values ≤ 5000 U/L, but it is mostly accompanied with underlying comorbid disorders such as acidosis, dehydration, as well as sepsis [9]. More details of association between AKI and rhabdomyolysis are described in chapter relating to renal manifestations of dengue infection.

Aggressive fluid resuscitation and alkalinization of the urine (sodium bicarbonate to increase urine pH > 6.5) are most important interventions. Urine alkalinization is performed with sodium bicarbonate to decrease myoglobin-induced nephrotoxicity in the tubules. Mannitol may also be prescribed to patients for prevention of renal complications. Since rhabdomyolysis may cause hyperkalemia due to massive release of intracellular potassium stores or AKI, appropriate measures should be carried out to correct the potassium levels in order to avoid any life-threatening complication [10]. Vigorous rehydration (both intravenously and orally), monitoring of fluid input and output charts, daily urinalyses for monitoring of pH, and close observation of laboratory indices including urea, creatinine, electrolytes, CPK, and platelet count are important considerations for the management of dengue-induced rhabdomyolysis [9].

7.3 Dengue-Induced Myalgia

Myalgia is characterized by pain, tenderness, and mild muscle swelling. Myalgia has been reported in up to 93% of dengue patients. Adult patients are more likely to have myalgia than pediatric patients. Moreover, the frequency of myalgia is also associated with the serotype of DENV, but the association of particular DENV with prevalence of myalgia is yet to be determined [1].

7.3.1 Clinical Manifestations of Dengue-Induced Myalgia

Diffuse myalgia is one of the classical symptoms of dengue fever and is observed during the starting point of the disease. Muscle pain frequently distresses the back and proximal limb muscles and might result in walking complications [7].

7.3.2 Pathogenesis of Dengue-Induced Myalgia

The exact pathogenesis of myalgia in dengue infection is not precisely known. Possibly, diffuse viral invasion of the muscles (at the time of viremia) and the resulting inflammatory variations in the muscles result in myalgia [1].

7.3.3 Diagnosis of Dengue-Induced Myalgia

Myalgia itself is a diagnostic tool of dengue and is usually ascertained with patient's complaints. Electromyography (EMG) is usually normal, but in patients with increased CK, mild myopathic changes have been recorded [14]. Other histopathological changes that can be seen included a mild to moderate perivascular mononuclear infiltrate, lipid accumulation, mild mitochondrial proliferation, few central nuclei, foci of muscle necrosis, and fiber type grouping [15].

7.3.4 Management of Dengue-Induced Myalgia

The dengue-induced myalgias are often transient and self-limiting. Severe muscle pain often responds to paracetamol.

7.4 Dengue-Induced Myositis

Myositis is defined as inflammation of skeletal muscles and is clinically characterized by pure motor weakness of all four limbs. Dengue-induced myositis can be of variable severity, ranging from self-limiting mild muscle weakness to severe dengue myositis that results in complete quadriplegia and respiratory insufficiency [16]. Myositis may concomitantly occur with myocarditis and is frequently associated with mortality [17]. Since etiology of myositis during dengue infection is based on neurological involvements, this complication is discussed in Chap. 6 (neurological complications of DVI).

7.4.1 Clinical Manifestations of Dengue-Induced Myositis

Myositis during the course of dengue infection is characterized by walking difficulties, muscle weakness, respiratory insufficiency, and quadriplegia [16].

7.4.2 Pathogenesis of Dengue-Induced Myositis

Direct viral invasion of the muscles possibly occurs during the acute stage of the illness. For example, the virus particles were found in the spleen, liver, and heart muscles after immediate intracerebral inoculation of dengue virus. In a study, DENV-2 was intracerebrally inoculated in adult Swiss albino mice. Electron microscopy revealed destruction of myofibrils, rarefaction of the sarcoplasmic reticulum network, and changes in the mitochondria. Aggregates of electron-dense material, as well as glycogen particles, were also seen in the cytoplasm [18]. As described previously, Salgado and co-workers have demonstrated the presence of DENV in postmortem samples of heart tissues of a patient with dengue virus myocarditis. These workers, in another set of in vitro experiments, demonstrated that human myoblasts infected with DENV caused an increased expression of the inflammatory genes and protein IP-10 (interferon gamma-induced protein 10) by the myotubes. In addition, the infected myotubes also had increased intracellular calcium levels [2]. Moreover,

DENV can infect muscle satellite cells; the main function of these cells is to repair muscles after injury. DVI is also responsible for causing impairment of dengue virus-infected muscle satellite cells to upregulate myosin heavy chain I protein levels, signifying that an immune reaction might be the reason of muscle damage [19].

7.4.3   Diagnosis of Dengue-Induced Myositis

High levels of CK are indicative of muscle inflammation. Other diagnostic tests may include determination of abnormal antibodies (to rule out any autoimmune disorder), MRI, and electromyography (EMG). EMG findings, in general, are consistent with the mild myopathic pattern. EMG usually reveals polyphasic and normal-to-short duration motor unit potentials, but spontaneous activity is absent. In addition, EMG can show early recruitment of motor unit action potentials with normal morphology [20]. Since Guillain–Barre syndrome is the most common referral indication, a differential diagnosis must be carried out [16]. In dengue-endemic areas, dengue myositis should be included in the differential diagnosis of pediatric acute flaccid paralysis. Dengue myositis in children is usually benign in nature. Dengue myositis is differentiated from other causes of walking difficulties by the presence of calf and thigh muscle tenderness on stretching, normal power and deep tendon reflexes, and an elevated CK [5, 15]. Muscle edema, hemorrhage, metabolic alterations, and changes in vascular endothelial cells are responsible for muscle dysfunction in dengue myositis. Cytokines, such as tumor necrosis factor, released during the viremia, lead to intense inflammation and subsequent damage to muscle fibers. Muscle histopathology, in these patients, revealed the presence of interstitial hemorrhage, myonecrosis, and myophagocytosis [5, 14].

7.4.4   Management of Dengue-Induced Myositis

Dengue-induced myositis usually resolves spontaneously, and most patients do not require any treatment. However, corticosteroids are used, but they have no definite role in resolution of myositis [1].

7.5   Dengue-Induced Osteonecrosis of Jaw

Osteonecrosis of the jaw (ONJ) is a severe bone disease (osteonecrosis) that affects the maxilla and the mandible region of the jaw. Various types of ONJ have been reported over the last decades, and a number of causes have been elaborated in the literature. Most of the reported cases of ONJ are associated with the use of bisphosphonates. Non-bisphosphonate causes include systemic medications such as steroids, antiangiogenic drugs, trauma, radiation, and chemicals such as formocresol used in dental treatment. The association of ONJ with bacterial, viral, and fungal infectious diseases is well established. Various infections such as noma, necrotizing ulcerative periodontitis, herpes zoster, aspergillosis, and mucormycosis have been found to be linked with the development of ONJ. ONJ can be graded into four stages based on the size of lesion. Identification of the underlying cause is really important for appropriate management [21]. Dengue-associated ONJ has been reported in the literature through individual case reports [22, 23].

7.5.1 Clinical Manifestations of Dengue-Induced Osteonecrosis of Jaw

Diffused erythematous swelling is usually associated with dengue-induced ONJ. Clinically ONJ is categorized into four severity stages ranging from Stage I to IV. Stage IV ONJ has been reported during the course of DVI. The differences in symptomology of these four stages are described below [23]:

- *Stage I*: The manifestation of exposed bone without any soft tissue infection. This stage is asymptomatic.
- *Stage II*: The presence of exposed bone with soft tissue infection. Patients in current stage of ONJ are usually symptomatic.
- *Stage III*: Patients are symptomatic with widespread exposed bone and soft tissue infection.
- *Stage IV*: There is extensive soft tissue infection along with hard tissue involvement. Patients are symptomatic in this stage.

7.5.2 Pathogenesis of Dengue-Induced Osteonecrosis of Jaw

As the life cycle of dengue virus begins, it has the tendency to enter blood stream and penetrate macrophages and monocytes which in turn enhances their ability to reproduce in the circulation [24]. The virus also activates CD4+ T cells. The monocytes release tumor necrosis factor-α which creates a cascade of cytokine activation, complement activation, and monocyte chemotactic protein-1 activation. The cytokine and chemokine cause leukopenia, increased vascular permeability, and thrombocytopenia and trigger coagulation and fibrinolysis [25]. Fibrinolysis and thrombocytopenia are factors that lead to hemorrhage and widespread capillary permeability causing edema and disseminated intravascular coagulopathy (DIC) and contribute to osteonecrosis. Complex cytokine interaction also causes bone marrow suppression and osteonecrosis [26]. Osteonecrosis could also be due to marrow suppression and intraosseous hemorrhage ultimately causing bone infarction and periodontal infection [21, 27]. One of the most characteristic clinical features that delineate osteomyelitis secondary to odontogenic and periodontal infection with ONJs in DVI is the absence of recession, mobility, attachment loss, and carious teeth. The proximity of the jaws to oral microorganisms could be one of the factors that predisposes jaws more than any other bone to develop osteonecrosis during the course of DVI.

7.5.3 Diagnosis of Dengue-Induced Osteonecrosis of Jaw

Intraoral examination is served to diagnose ONJ. Patients may have complete gingival recession with irregular exposure of alveolar bone and a part of basal bone in both the left and the right maxillary quadrants extending from lateral incisors to the first molar. Moreover, patients might have evident root pieces. Orthopantomogram can reveal irregular radiolucency that involves both alveolar and basal bone in both maxillary quadrants in the region of lateral incisor and the second molar. Bone destruction can be observed using cone beam computed tomography and contrast-enhanced computed tomography. Since there are many other etiological factors precipitating ONJ, differential diagnosis is of utmost importance for optimal treatment. There are many pathological conditions which share similar clinical manifestations as of ONJ. Chronic suppurative osteomyelitis and noma are two important diseases which should be subjected to differential diagnosis. Noma (cancrum oris) is an orofacial gangrene, which causes progressive and disfiguring destruction of the infected tissues. ONJ can be differentiated from chronic suppurative osteomyelitis based on the primary etiology. The major differences and similarities between ONJ, osteomyelitis, and noma are presented in Table 7.1.

7.5.4 Management of Dengue-Induced Osteonecrosis of Jaw

ONJs are generally managed conservatively. Evidences have shown considerable improvements in disease prognosis through conservative measures as given below:

- Optimal oral hygiene
- Treatment and eradication of active dental and periodontal disease
- Mouth rinsing and gargling with topical antibiotics
- Systemic antibiotic course, if prescribed

Conservative management remains the mainstay of patient's care with ONJ. It must be noted that conservative measures may not necessarily resolve the lesions completely. However, patients may improve symptomatically and have long-term relief with these measures. Surgery is an option for nonresponsive ONJ cases. Ostectomy is a type of surgical procedure of the infected area with resection margins that extend into adjacent normal-appearing bone. Moreover, management of ONJ depends upon the stage of the disease. The management of ONJ according to its state is described below [23]:

- *Stage I*: The management of this stage is recommended via mouth rinsing with chlorhexidine (twice daily).
- *Stage II*: Chlorhexidine mouth rinses plus antibiotics and analgesics.
- *Stage III*: Soft tissue debridement is performed along with chlorhexidine mouth rinses.
- *Stage IV*: Soft and hard tissue debridement is performed followed by antibiotics and analgesics.

Table 7.1 Differential diagnosis of ONJ from chronic suppurative osteomyelitis and noma

ONJ and chronic suppurative osteomyelitis	
ONJ	**Chronic suppurative osteomyelitis**
Avascular necrosis of jaw bones	Infection of medullary portion of jaw bones
Absence of involucrum and sequestrum formation	Involucrum and sequestrum formation are present
Presence of necrotic bone with empty lacunae	Presence of necrotic bone with empty lacunae
No inflammatory infiltrate in marrow tissues	Marked degree of inflammatory infiltrate in marrow tissues
Remodeling of the bone is absent	Remodeling of bone is present
ONJ and noma	
ONJ	**Noma**
ONJ is not primarily an infection	Noma is an infectious condition which is more prevalent among immunocompromised people and malnourished children with poor oral hygiene. *Prevotella intermedia* and *Fusobacterium necrophorum* are the most common pathogens underlying the noma
There is no cutaneous involvement in ONJ	Cutaneous involvement has been observed in noma, as dermonecrotic toxins are produced by *Fusobacterium necrophorum*
Absence of gangrenous involvement of tissues	Presence of gangrenous involvement of tissues
There is no discoloration of tissues in ONJ	Blackish discoloration of tissues has been observed clinically

Table is self-constructed. Information is extracted from two sources [28, 29]

7.6   Dengue-Induced Hypokalemic Paralysis

Hypokalemic paralysis responsive to oral or intravenous potassium supplementation has been well documented during the course of DVI. The exact mechanism responsible for hypokalemic paralysis is not known. Redistribution of potassium ions in the cells and transient renal tubular abnormalities are major postulated pathogeneses of hypokalemia during DVI. Both these processes cause increased urinary potassium wasting among patients. Elevated levels of catecholamine and secondary insulin release possibly trigger the redistribution of potassium in the cells. The reported prevalence of dengue-associated hypokalemia is around 70%, but patients seldom develop paralysis. However, the role of genetic susceptibility cannot be disregarded. Mutations in two skeletal muscle genes are associated with hypokalemic periodic paralysis among patients. Mutations in the alpha subunit of the L-type calcium channel gene (CACNA14) contribute majorly in the development of hypokalemic periodic paralysis, while mutations in the alpha subunit of the sodium channel gene (SCN4A) in association with paralysis have been observed in few cases. It is probable that dengue-associated hypokalemic paralysis represents some kind of channelopathy [30]. Clinical manifestations, diagnosis, and management of this complication are provided in Chap. 6.

7.7   Dengue-Induced Post-Infectious Fatigue Syndrome

Post-infectious fatigue syndrome is defined as persisting fatigue and disability after apparent acute infections. Fatigue syndrome has been reported in up to 3.2% cases after dengue infection. Moreover, extended fatigue syndrome is also reported after DVI. Existing data suggest advanced age, female gender, the manifestation of chills, and the lack of rashes are suggestively associated with the development of fatigue in post-dengue infection [1, 31].

The exact mechanism of fatigue after the dengue infection has not been precisely postulated in literature. Post-infectious fatigue syndrome is possibly a consequence of systemic immune alterations (triggered by the DENV). It has also been postulated that interactions of the immunological, endocrinal, musculoskeletal, and neurological systems, possibly via hypothalamic–pituitary–adrenal axis and the autonomic nervous system, resulting in fatigue syndrome [31].

7.8   Dengue Infection with Myasthenia Gravis

Myasthenia gravis (MG) is a very common immune-mediated neuromuscular junction disease which is primarily characterized by fluctuating motor weakness. Ocular and bulbar musculatures are primarily involved in the clinical manifestations of MG. Circulating antibodies against postsynaptic acetylcholine receptors are cardinal feature of MG. MG is accompanied by a wide range of clinical manifestations as described below [32]:

- Fatigue
- Diplopia
- Ptosis
- Dysphagia
- Difficulty in mastication
- Dysarthria
- Proximal and neck muscle weakness
- Acute respiratory insufficiency due to involvement of respiratory muscles

The diagnosis of MG is essentially based on laboratory tests and the presence of antibodies among patients. The presence of serum acetylcholine receptor antibodies, positive edrophonium test, and decreased activity on repetitive nerve stimulation are some important diagnostic implications for MG [33]. Patients with MG may progress to myasthenic crisis or cholinergic crisis. Both these conditions require ICU admission [34].

7.8.1 Myasthenic Crisis and Its Management

Myasthenic crisis (MC) is defined as respiratory weakness in patients with acquired, autoimmune form of MG. The lifelong risk of MC in patients with MG is about 20–30%. The occurrence of myasthenic crisis varies according to the age. Among young patients, it is frequently observed during the early course of symptomatic disease, while it occurs late among elderly patients with MG. The management of myasthenic crisis is well established. Intubation and mechanical ventilation are used in most of the patients who developed myasthenic crisis. Moreover, immunosuppression along with acetylcholinesterase inhibitors is a promising treatment for such patients [35, 36]. Pyridostigmine is the most widely used symptomatic drug in MG. Neostigmine is also used in these patients and has advantage of fast onset of action. The first-choice immunosuppressants are prednisolone and azathioprine. There are numerous second-line medications for MG including cyclosporine, methotrexate, and mycophenolate mofetil. Thymectomy is reserved for patients having MG concomitantly with thymoma and for those with early-onset MG. IV immunoglobulin and plasma exchange are equally effective and safe therapeutic modalities for MG crisis and other acute exacerbations [35, 36].

7.8.2 Cholinergic Crisis

Cholinergic crisis is secondary to excess cholinesterase inhibitor medication. In patients with cholinergic crisis, excessive acetylcholinergic stimulation of striated muscles at the neuromuscular junction results in flaccid muscle paralysis that can be difficult to differentiate from weakness due to myasthenia crisis. The differential diagnosis of cholinergic versus myasthenic crisis always remains a challenge for physicians as both conditions present with respiratory failure. Cholinergic crisis is classically manifested as decreased blood pressure, abdominal cramps, nausea, vomiting, diarrhea, blurred vision, pallor, facial muscle twitching, constriction of pupils, and no effect with Tensilon test. Patients with cholinergic crisis demonstrate improved symptoms with the administration of anticholinergics, i.e., atropine. However, in certain clinical conditions, if it is very challenging to differentiate myasthenic and cholinergic crisis, acetylcholinesterase inhibitor therapy must be terminated in such cases, and the patient should be monitored in ICU [35].

7.8.3 Dengue Infection and Myasthenia Gravis

DVI has been reported to cause worsening of muscle weakness in patients with MG. However, symptoms subsequently improve with the resolution of dengue infection. Available literature indicates that patients with stable MG and on pyridostigmine therapy may experience muscle weakness of similar severity which is present at the time of diagnosis of MG [37]. However, it must be noted that symptoms of MG can also be effected by various other clinical features such as emotional distress, systemic diseases (mainly viral respiratory infections), thyroid gland dysfunction (both hypothyroidism and hyperthyroidism), pregnancy, menstrual cycle, hyper pyrexia, and drugs affecting neuromuscular transmission [38]. Myalgia or myositis symptoms such as muscle ache and hypokalemia are not observed among patients. Pyridostigmine along with vigorous fluid replacement may provide improvement in symptoms [37].

DVI-associated myasthenic crisis has been reported in patient with MG [39]. It is possible that the neurotropic effect of the DENV causes progressive worsening of the weakness in the early incubation period which eventually leads to the respiratory failure resulting in myasthenic crisis during the febrile phase of the dengue infection. However, clinicians must also consider noncompliance as a risk factor of myasthenic crisis. IVIg and plasma exchange have shown promising benefits to the patients with myasthenic crisis [34].

7.9   Dengue-Induced Arthralgia

Rheumatic manifestations like joint pains are the most important clinical characteristics of dengue, although often overshadowed by other symptoms such as biphasic fever, skin rash, conjunctival suffusion, pharyngitis, headache, abdominal pain, vomiting, photophobia, orbital pain, and hemorrhagic manifestations [40]. About two-third of individuals with DVI suffer from joint pain, with preponderance of peripheral joints. Active synovitis like effusion and morning stiffness has not been described during the course of DVI [41]. The incidence of joint pain is much higher in adults as compared to children. It must be noted that severity of pain in joints does not relate with the severity of dengue infection [42].

Since many other viral infections including chikungunya, Ross River fever, Sindbis virus infection, Pogosta fever, and Mayaro fever are associated with arthralgia, clinicians must carry out differential diagnosis to rule out the exact cause of the pain. Joint pains with effusions are primarily associated with chikungunya, while all other infections are linked with persistent or recurrent arthralgia [43, 44]. Treatment of joint pains is purely symptomatic. Because of associated thrombocytopenia, NSAIDs should be avoided. However paracetamol can be given safely. Arthralgia possesses excellent prognosis and disappears after DVI in most of the patients. However, the presence of arthralgia after 2 years of dengue infection has been reported in 29.5% patients in a study. Authors have described changes in a few immunological factors and FcγRIIa gene polymorphism as possible contributor of persisting symptoms. These findings suggest that autoimmune-based disturbance may relate to clinical sequelae even after 2 years of recovery from an acute DVI [45].

7.10 Dengue Infection in Patients with Lupus and Rheumatoid Arthritis

Lupus is an autoimmune disease, also termed as systemic lupus erythematosus (SLE). In this disease, the immune system erroneously assaults healthy tissues of the body. It can affect all major organs of the body including the skin, joints, kidneys, brain, and other organs. Rheumatoid arthritis (RA) is a long-standing autoimmune disorder that mainly affects joints. These rheumatic disorders may contribute to severe outcome of DVI. Existing data indicate that outline of DVI among rheumatologic disease patients may be different from that in general population. Patients with DVI along with RA or SLE portend substantial morbidity, mortality, and increased hospitalization [46]. Clinicians must prioritize the dengue care in patient with preexisting rheumatic diseases.

7.11 Dengue-Induced Sacroiliitis

There is lack of evidence on arthritogenic nature of dengue virus. Dengue-associated sacroiliitis has been reported in young female and pregnant women [47, 48]. Sacroiliitis may occur as a separate disease entity due to infectious disease or as part of an inflammatory arthropathy such as seronegative spondyloarthropathy. Brucellosis and tuberculosis are two frequently prevailed bacterial infections having predilection for sacroiliac joints. Both these infections cause unilateral sacroiliac disease. The occurrence non-brucellosis and non-tuberculous infective sacroiliitis is quite rare. Among other bacterial causes of sacroiliitis, staphylococci and *Pseudomonas aeruginosa* are frequently identified among cases [49]. There are also several reports of viral arthritides. Viruses itself in the form of infection or as cofactor can cause the development of rheumatic diseases. There is a broad list of viruses causing arthritis including rubella, mumps, parvovirus B19, hepatitis B virus, hepatitis C virus, Epstein–Barr virus, cytomegalovirus, and the group of arthritogenic alphaviruses. Arthritogenic alphaviruses have potential to predispose bone abnormalities during the course of infection. Chikungunya virus, Ross River virus (RRV), Barmah Forest virus, Sindbis virus, o'nyong-nyong virus, and Mayaro virus are some common examples of arthritogenic alphaviruses [50]. A prime attention must be paid to the differential diagnosis among dengue patients. Moreover, sensible way to exclude the septic arthritis is a mainstay of the treatment.

Several hypotheses underlying the pathogenesis of viral arthritis exist in the literature [47]. The following is the list of well-direct well-established mechanisms of virus-associated arthritis:

• Attack of the synovium and the joint tissue due to viral tropism for the synovial tissue
• Formation and subsequent deposition of immune complexes in the joint tissue as the viral particles act as antigenic components

- Immune dysregulation
- Virus-induced autoimmunity

The high levels of inflammatory cytokine including interleukin-6 (IL-6), enhanced receptor activator of nuclear factor kappa-B ligand (RANKL), and decreased osteoprotegerin (OPG) cause osteoclasts to increase in bone reabsorption and bone pathologies. In this context, anti-IL-6R antibodies (i.e., tocilizumab) at earlier stages will provide therapeutic benefits. Moreover, inhibition of IL-6 improves the inflammation and is also considered as an effective therapeutic approach in such cases [51]. DENV may share similar pathological mechanisms to induce arthritis. It has been hypothesized that DENV induces IL-6, hence following the similar cascade as described. There is no recommended management therapy for dengue-induced sacroiliitis, and symptomatic treatment with analgesics is considered sufficient. Though it has been hypothesized that DENV might cause or exaggerate sacroiliitis, there is also a high propensity that the sacroiliitis merely coincides with the DVI. In this regard, more histopathological investigations are needed to ascertain the exact relationship between DENV and sacroiliitis and other forms of arthritis [47].

7.12 Dengue-Induced Bone Marrow Suppression

The bone marrow (BM) has either direct or indirect involvement in dengue pathogenesis. Several investigations conducted on the BM cells demonstrate that patients with DVI have early BM suppression as a common clinical feature [52]. The evidence of DENV in BM has been found through autopsy findings where virus is identified in BM of DSS fatal cases and in BM of DHF survived cases [53]. BM-related aplasia is infrequent presentation during DVI but has been documented in the literature [54]. Findings from experimental studies elaborate that DENV can proficiently infect hematopoietic cells [55]. These studies underscore that DENV replicates only in leukocytes which are derived from the BM and does not replicate in leukocytes derived from other lymphatic tissues such as spleen, thymus, and lymph node [56]. These findings in humans are in concordance with the results derived from studies conducted in monkeys where BM was observed to be an early target of DENV replication [57]. Though the evidence of BM involvement during DVI is well established in previous studies, the role of the BM as a site for DENV replication is not validated. It might be due to the reason that BM biopsies from dengue patients are quite difficult due to the increased risk of bleeding during the procedure [58].

A study on primate animal model indicates the potential contribution of megakaryocytes in the BM compartment to the life cycle of DENV infection [58]. However, the results of this study must be carefully interpreted. Since megakaryocytes have various features that are similar to hematopoietic stem cells, there might be a possibility that the cells observed in this study are hematopoietic stem cells

[59]. Nevertheless, the role of these cells is yet to be elucidated. These cells either disseminate virus to other parts of the body or play a crucial part in virus replication, transmission, and disease pathogenesis. The exact mechanism through which these cells involve in the course of DVI needs to be delineated. Findings of this study provide evidence that systemic infection of nonhuman primate with DENV causes direct infection of BM, which leads to transient cell suppression in the peripheral blood [58].

BM demonstrates hypocellularity and attenuation of megakaryocyte maturation during the early phase of the disease. DENV-associated BM suppression during the acute phase of DVI can be caused by various mechanisms involving the three main contributors:

1. DENV-induced direct lesion of progenitor cells
2. Infection of stromal cells
3. Alterations in bone marrow regulation

Megakaryocytopoiesis and platelet production in human is regulated by a cytokine "thrombopoietin (TPO)." It regulates blood cell production through activating TPO receptor c-MPL (myeloproliferative leukemia virus oncogene). Since the levels of TPO elevate during the decrease production of platelets, serum TPO levels might be served as a beneficial tool of megakaryocytopoiesis among patients with DVI. Recent findings have indicated significantly lower TPO levels in adult DVI patients having substantial reduction of thrombocytes. Similarly, lower levels of TPO in human serum suggest markedly improved or higher platelet counts [60].

References

1. Garg RK, Malhotra HS, Jain A, Malhotra KP. Dengue-associated neuromuscular complications. Neurol India. 2015;63(4):497.
2. Salgado DM, Eltit JM, Mansfield K, Panqueba C, Castro D, Vega MR, et al. Heart and skeletal muscle are targets of dengue virus infection. Pediatr Infect Dis J. 2010;29(3):238.
3. Gulati S, Maheshwari A. Atypical manifestations of dengue. Tropical Med Int Health. 2007;12(9):1087–95.
4. Sani SSM, Han WH, Bujang MA, Ding HJ, Ng KL, Shariffuddin MAA. Evaluation of creatine kinase and liver enzymes in identification of severe dengue. BMC Infect Dis. 2017;17(1):505.
5. Kalita J, Misra U, Mahadevan A, Shankar S. Acute pure motor quadriplegia: is it dengue myositis? Electromyogr Clin Neurophysiol. 2005;45(6):357–61.
6. Misra U, Kalita J, Syam U, Dhole T. Neurological manifestations of dengue virus infection. J Neurol Sci. 2006;244(1–2):117–22.
7. Finsterer J, Kongchan K. Severe, persisting, steroid-responsive dengue myositis. J Clin Virol. 2006;35(4):426–8.
8. Bosch X, Poch E, Grau JM. Rhabdomyolysis and acute kidney injury. N Engl J Med. 2009;361(1):62–72.
9. Sargeant T, Harris T, Wilks R, Barned S, Galloway-Blake K, Ferguson T. Rhabdomyolysis and dengue fever: a case report and literature review. Case Rep Med. 2013;2013:101058.
10. Cervellin G, Comelli I, Lippi G. Rhabdomyolysis: historical background, clinical, diagnostic and therapeutic features. Clin Chem Lab Med. 2010;48(6):749–56.

11. Repizo LP, Malheiros DM, Yu L, Barros RT, Burdmann EA. Biopsy proven acute tubular necrosis due to rhabdomyolysis in a dengue fever patient: a case report and review of literature. Rev Inst Med Trop Sao Paulo. 2014;56(1):85–8.
12. Davis JS, Bourke P. Rhabdomyolysis associated with dengue virus infection. Clin Infect Dis. 2004;38(10):e109–e11.
13. Gagnon SJ, Mori M, Kurane I, Green S, Vaughn DW, Kalayanarooj S, et al. Cytokine gene expression and protein production in peripheral blood mononuclear cells of children with acute dengue virus infections. J Med Virol. 2002;67(1):41–6.
14. Misra U, Kalita J, Maurya P, Kumar P, Shankar S, Mahadevan A. Dengue-associated transient muscle dysfunction: clinical, electromyography and histopathological changes. Infection. 2012;40(2):125–30.
15. Malheiros SMF, Oliveira ASB, Schmidt B, Lima J, Gabbai AA. Dengue: muscle biopsy findings in 15 patients. Arq Neuropsiquiatr. 1993;51(2):159–64.
16. Paliwal VK, Garg RK, Juyal R, Husain N, Verma R, Sharma PK, et al. Acute dengue virus myositis: a report of seven patients of varying clinical severity including two cases with severe fulminant myositis. J Neurol Sci. 2011;300(1–2):14–8.
17. Sangle SA, Dasgupta A, Ratnalikar SD, Kulkarni RV. Dengue myositis and myocarditis. Neurol India. 2010;58(4):598.
18. Nath P, Agrawal DK, Mehrotra R. Ultrastructural changes in skeletal muscles in dengue virus-infected mice. J Pathol. 1982;136(4):301–5.
19. Warke RV, Becerra A, Zawadzka A, Schmidt DJ, Martin KJ, Giaya K, et al. Efficient dengue virus (DENV) infection of human muscle satellite cells upregulates type I interferon response genes and differentially modulates MHC I expression on bystander and DENV-infected cells. J Gen Virol. 2008;89(7):1605–15.
20. Rajajee S, Ezhilarasi S, Rajarajan K. Benign acute childhood myositis. Indian J Pediatr. 2005;72(5):399–400.
21. Almazrooa SA, Woo S-B. Bisphosphonate and nonbisphosphonate-associated osteonecrosis of the jaw: a review. J Am Dent Assoc. 2009;140(7):864–75.
22. Prakash SR, Nasim A, Kamarthi N, Gupta S. Osteonecrosis of jaw bones: a complication of severe dengue. J Indian Acad Oral Med Radiol. 2018;30(2):173.
23. Patil PP, Bhavthankar JD, Mandale MS, Humbe JG. Jaw osteonecrosis preceded by dengue fever-possible pathogenetic mechanism. J Orthop Case Rep. 2018;8(6):9.
24. Chaturvedi U, Dhawan R, Khanna M, Mathur A. Breakdown of the blood-brain barrier during dengue virus infection of mice. J Gen Virol. 1991;72(4):859–66.
25. Dubey P, Kumar S, Bansal V, Kumar KA, Mowar A, Khare G. Postextraction bleeding following a fever: a case report. Oral Surg Oral Med Oral Pathol Oral Radiol. 2013;115(1):e27–31.
26. Chuansumrit A, Chaiyaratana W. Hemostatic derangement in dengue hemorrhagic fever. Thromb Res. 2014;133(1):10–6.
27. Khan AA, Morrison A, Hanley DA, Felsenberg D, McCauley LK, O'Ryan F, et al. Diagnosis and management of osteonecrosis of the jaw: a systematic review and international consensus. J Bone Miner Res. 2015;30(1):3–23.
28. Tolstunov L, Cox D, Javid B. Odontogenic osteomyelitis or bisphosphonate-related osteonecrosis of mandible of patient with autoimmune disease: clinical dilemma. Compend Contin Educ Dent. 2012;33(10):E116–22.
29. Enwonwu C, Falkler W Jr, Idigbe E. Oro-facial gangrene (noma/cancrum oris): pathogenetic mechanisms. Crit Rev Oral Biol Med. 2000;11(2):159–71.
30. Malhotra HS, Garg RK. Dengue-associated hypokalemic paralysis: causal or incidental? J Neurol Sci. 2014;340(1-2):19–25.
31. Seet RC, Quek AM, Lim EC. Post-infectious fatigue syndrome in dengue infection. J Clin Virol. 2007;38(1):1–6.
32. Conti-Fine BM, Milani M, Kaminski HJ. Myasthenia gravis: past, present, and future. J Clin Invest. 2006;116(11):2843–54.
33. Benatar M. A systematic review of diagnostic studies in myasthenia gravis. Neuromuscul Disord. 2006;16(7):459–67.

34. Chaudhuri A, Behan P. Myasthenic crisis. QJM. 2008;102(2):97–107.
35. Juel VC, editor. Myasthenia gravis: management of myasthenic crisis and perioperative care. Semin Neurol. 2004;24(1):75–81.
36. Jani-Acsadi A, Lisak RP. Myasthenic crisis: guidelines for prevention and treatment. J Neurol Sci. 2007;261(1–2):127–33.
37. Hardjo Lugito N, Margaret AK. Worsening muscle weakness in myasthenia gravis patient suffering dengue infection. J Trop Dis Public Health. 2014;2:3.
38. Gilhus NE, Verschuuren JJ. Myasthenia gravis: subgroup classification and therapeutic strategies. Lancet Neurol. 2015;14(10):1023–36.
39. Thabit AAM, Kamil WMRWA, Din MRM. Dengue fever in myasthenic crisis. Int J Trop Dis Health. 2016;18(4):1–5.
40. Harris E, Videa E, Pérez L, Sandoval E, Téllez Y, Perez M, et al. Clinical, epidemiologic, and virologic features of dengue in the 1998 epidemic in Nicaragua. Am J Trop Med Hyg. 2000;63(1):5–11.
41. Adebajo A. Dengue arthritis. Rheumatology. 1996;35(9):909–10.
42. Phuong CXT, Nhan NT, Kneen R, Thuy PTT, Van Thien C, Nga NTT, et al. Clinical diagnosis and assessment of severity of confirmed dengue infections in Vietnamese children: is the World Health Organization classification system helpful? Am J Trop Med Hyg. 2004;70(2):172–9.
43. Laine M, Luukkainen R, Toivanen A. Sindbis viruses and other alphaviruses as cause of human arthritic disease. J Intern Med. 2004;256(6):457–71.
44. Mylonas AD, Brown AM, Carthew TL, Purdie DM, Pandeya N, Collins LG, et al. Natural history of Ross River virus-induced epidemic polyarthritis. Med J Aust. 2002;177(7):356–60.
45. García G, González N, Pérez AB, Sierra B, Aguirre E, Rizo D, et al. Long-term persistence of clinical symptoms in dengue-infected persons and its association with immunological disorders. Int J Infect Dis. 2011;15(1):e38–43.
46. de Abreu MM, Maiorano AC, Tedeschi SK, Yoshida K, Lin T-C, Solomon DH, editors. Outcomes of lupus and rheumatoid arthritis patients with primary dengue infection: a seven-year report from Brazil. Semin Arthritis Rheum. 2018;47(5):749–55.
47. Jayamali W, Herath H, Kulatunga A. A young female presenting with unilateral sacroiliitis following dengue virus infection: a case report. J Med Case Rep. 2017;11(1):307.
48. Umakanth M. Dengue complicated with sacroiliitis in a pregnant woman. Int J Health Sci Res. 2018;8(7):333–76.
49. Hermet M, Minichiello E, Flipo RM, Dubost JJ, Allanore Y, Ziza JM, et al. Infectious sacroiliitis: a retrospective, multicentre study of 39 adults. BMC Infect Dis. 2012;12(1):305.
50. Smith J, Chalupa P, Hasan MS. Infectious arthritis: clinical features, laboratory findings and treatment. Clin Microbiol Infect. 2006;12(4):309–14.
51. Chen W, Foo S-S, Rulli NE, Taylor A, Sheng K-C, Herrero LJ, et al. Arthritogenic alphaviral infection perturbs osteoblast function and triggers pathologic bone loss. Proc Natl Acad Sci. 2014;111(16):6040–5.
52. Bierman HR, Nelson ER. Hematodepressive virus diseases of Thailand. Ann Intern Med. 1965;62(5):867–84.
53. Nisalak A, Halstead S, Singharaj P, Udomsakdi S, Nye S, Vinijchaikul K. Observations related to pathogenesis of dengue hemorrhagic fever. 3. Virologic studies of fatal disease. Yale J Biol Med. 1970;42(5):293.
54. Srichaikul T, Punyagupta S, Kanchanapoom T, Chanokovat C, Likittanasombat K, Leelasiri A. Hemophagocytic syndrome in dengue hemorrhagic fever with severe multiorgan complications. J Med Assoc Thail. 2008;91(1):104–9.
55. Bente DA, Melkus MW, Garcia JV, Rico-Hesse R. Dengue fever in humanized NOD/SCID mice. J Virol. 2005;79(21):13797–9.
56. Halstead S, O'rourke E, Allison A. Dengue viruses and mononuclear phagocytes. II. Identity of blood and tissue leukocytes supporting in vitro infection. J Exp Med. 1977;146(1):218–29.
57. La Russa VF, Innis BL. 11 mechanisms of dengue virus-induced bone marrow suppression. Baillières Clin Haematol. 1995;8(1):249–70.

58. Noisakran S, Onlamoon N, Hsiao H-M, Clark KB, Villinger F, Ansari AA, et al. Infection of bone marrow cells by dengue virus in vivo. Exp Hematol. 2012;40(3):250–9. e4.
59. Huang H, Cantor AB. Common features of megakaryocytes and hematopoietic stem cells: what's the connection? J Cell Biochem. 2009;107(5):857–64.
60. de Azeredo EL, Monteiro RQ, de Oliveira Pinto LM. Thrombocytopenia in dengue: interrelationship between virus and the imbalance between coagulation and fibrinolysis and inflammatory mediators. Mediat Inflamm. 2015;2015:313842.

Dengue-Induced Lymphoreticular Complications

8

8.1 Lymphoreticular Involvements in Dengue Infection

Dengue virus (DENV) has been predominantly found in the cells of the spleen, thymus, and lymph nodes. Lymphadenopathy, also known as adenopathy, is observed in half of the DHF cases, while it is rarely reported in small infants. Lymph node infarcts and splenic rupture are unusual but fatal complications of DHF [1, 2]. DENV causes substantial histopathological alternations in the tissues of the immune system including atrophy and depletion of cells in the periarterial lymphatic sheaths of the spleen and the paracortical areas of the lymph nodes, hypoplasia of the bone marrow, acute atrophy, and wasting of the thymus. Thymus-dependent areas of the spleen and lymph nodes are primarily affected as compared to thymus-independent areas of the secondary lymphatic tissues [3]. Following lymphoreticular complications have been observed during the course of dengue viral infection (DVI).

1. Splenic rupture
2. Lymphadenopathy
3. Splenomegaly
4. Lymph node infarction

8.2 Dengue-Induced Splenic Rupture

The spleen is a delicate structure in the human body that is located in the upper left abdomen. Its prime functions are blood filtration, recycling of red blood cells, storage of platelets and white blood cells, and thus fight against certain kinds of bacteria [4]. Splenic rupture is a potentially fatal disorder and is often associated with chest or abdominal trauma. Spontaneous rupture is very rare and is frequently associated with underlying hematological, neoplastic, inflammatory, and infectious disorders [5]. Splenic rupture can be posttraumatic or nontraumatic (atraumatic). Posttraumatic splenic rupture is a common condition, while nontraumatic is rare. Nontraumatic

© Springer Nature Singapore Pte Ltd. 2021
T. H. Mallhi et al., *Expanded Dengue Syndrome*,
https://doi.org/10.1007/978-981-15-7337-8_8

splenic rupture may have some pathology or can occur spontaneously. Splenic disease is an important factor of pathological nontraumatic splenic rupture that manifests itself with abnormal histology, whereas there is no evidence of histological changes in case of spontaneous nontraumatic rupture [6]. Nontraumatic splenic rupture may result from infections (malaria, mononucleosis, dengue, typhoid, aspergillosis, endocarditis), malignancy (non-Hodgkin's lymphoma, myeloid leukemia, chronic lymphocytic leukemia, metastases of various tumors), or connective tissue disease. Hematologic malignancies such as choriocarcinoma, teratoma, and malignant melanoma are predominant causes of splenic rupture. Some rare disorders including polyarteritis nodosa, collagenosis, systemic lupus erythematosus (SLE), and granulomatosis are also linked with splenic rupture [7].

Spontaneous splenic rupture is a rare but documented complication of both DF and DHF [8]. In severe dengue, the spleen is frequently congested, and autopsy reveals subcapsular hematomas in approximately 15% of examined cases. Contrary to severe dengue, splenic rupture is extremely rare in dengue infection, and merely a few cases have been reported [8]. Spontaneous splenic rupture usually occurs during the early course of dengue illness, but it can also prevail during the recovery phase of infection [9].

8.2.1 Pathogenesis of Splenic Rupture During Dengue Infection

The pathophysiological mechanism underpinning dengue-associated splenic rupture is not yet well elucidated, but it is reported to be caused by deficiency of coagulation factors and platelets that results in intrasplenic hemorrhage that ultimately leads to splenic rupture [10]. The widely acknowledged hypothesis suggests that splenic rupture is mainly caused by subcapsular hemorrhage that occurs as a result of various vascular abnormalities, reduced coagulation factors, and fatal thrombocytopenia [7, 11]. In majority of dengue infection cases, splenic rupture manifests itself in the viremic phase of infection, before development of antibodies. However, splenic rupture during recovery phase of dengue infection has been reported in literature [9]. The prevalent case of splenic rupture during the recovery phase contradicts the aforementioned theory related to the pathogenesis of dengue-induced splenic rupture. It is evident that coagulation profile and platelet count improve during the dengue recovery phase; thus, splenic rupture in this phase might be attributed to another cause. A possible mechanism might be severe splenic congestion leading to laceration and subcapsular hematoma formation [9].

8.2.2 Clinical Manifestations of Dengue-Induced Splenic Rupture

The most frequent clinical manifestation of splenic rupture includes abdominal pain. Diffused pain followed by pain in the upper left abdomen are classical characteristics of abdominal pain in splenic rupture. In many cases, this pain evolves to peritoneal irritation in association with hemorrhagic shock signs (tachycardia, hypotension, and reduced hematocrit). Acute acalculous cholecystitis, differential diagnosis for splenic rupture, is a well-established complication of dengue that is also presented with abdominal pain. The abdominal pain caused by acute acalculous cholecystitis prevails in the upper right abdomen with a positive Murphy signal, with or without extravasation shock signs. The common extravasation clinical signs in severe dengue (hypotension, tachycardia, and oliguria) might also indicate a splenic rupture bleeding [5, 10]. Both splenic rupture-associated shock and classic dengue shock can be easily misdiagnosed since both shocks develop hypotension and tachycardia. The distinguishing feature between both shocks is hematocrit value. The hematocrit value decreases in splenic rupture shock while increases in dengue shock syndrome (DSS).

8.2.3 Diagnosis of Dengue-Induced Splenic Rupture

There are various diagnostic techniques for splenic rupture. Paracentesis is an effective diagnostic test that is carried out to detect spontaneous splenic rupture and suspected intraperitoneal and unstable hemorrhage [6]. For rapid diagnosis of both intraperitoneal fluid and blood, ultrasonography is an inexpensive test frequently employed in the emergency department. Computed tomography (CT) detects splenic rupture as well as severity of the splenic lesion and additionally provides information regarding free fluid in the abdominal cavity. Considering the effectiveness, noninvasive nature, and lack of associated risks, ultrasonography is suitable for patients with hemodynamic instabilities. On the other hand, diagnostic measure such as CT is beneficial for hemodynamically stable patients [5, 6, 12].

The histopathological examinations of patients show lymphoid follicles and proteins in macrophages and endothelial cells [10]. It must be noted that splenic histology might be normal in some cases [13].

8.2.4 Management of Dengue-Induced Splenic Rupture

The management of spontaneous splenic rupture is well documented. The treatments revolve around conservation or surgical removal of spleen (splenectomy). Existing data indicate survival rate of pathological splenic rupture as 63% with splenectomy and only 7% with conservative measures [14]. Surgical treatment of spontaneous splenic rupture controls bleeding, rectifies thrombocytopenia, and reestablishes hemostasis in approximately 2 days. The use of recombinant factor VIIa has also been reported in pediatric population in order to avoid surgery. However, the use of factor is accompanied by few shortcomings including high cost and lack of clinical evidence from randomized clinical trials. It is suggested that factor VIIa should be reserved for extreme circumstances where risks of surgical intervention outweighs the risk of massive thrombosis [13]. The current recommendations still recommends splenectomy in majority of dengue infection cases.

However, satisfactory results have been reported with conservative treatment in non-severe dengue patients [6, 11]. In conclusion, the correct therapeutic choice for dengue-induced splenic rupture is governed by the hemodynamic status of the patient.

8.3   Dengue-Induced Lymphadenopathy

Lymphadenopathy refers to the abnormal enlargement of lymph nodes. Dengue-induced lymphadenopathy is generally not a feature of dengue infection, but it has been reported among 40–50% of dengue cases [15, 16].

8.3.1   Pathogenesis of Dengue-Induced Lymphadenopathy

The exact pathogenesis of lymphadenopathy during the course of dengue infection is not clear. However, the presence of virus in the lymph nodes is well documented [17].

8.3.2   Clinical Manifestations of Dengue-Induced Lymphadenopathy

Dengue-induced lymphadenopathy presents with painless and enlarged lymph nodes on the groin, head, or neck region.

8.3.3   Diagnosis of Dengue-Induced Lymphadenopathy

Dengue-induced lymphadenopathy is diagnosed through physical examination of patients. Lymph node enlargement is usually defined as a node size of more than 1 cm. Complete blood count aids in diagnostic workup of patients. In a few cases, a biopsy of the gland is needed if the cause of lymph enlargement is unknown. Complicated lymphadenopathy is indicated by protracted enlargement of the lymph nodes thus hinting directly at lymphomas; biopsy is done in such cases [1, 12].

8.3.4   Management of Dengue-Induced Lymphadenopathy

There is practically no treatment of dengue-induced lymphadenopathy. The management of such patients aims to minimize the symptoms and includes sufficient bed rest, adequate use of analgesics, and excessive water intake. Treatment is determined by the specific underlying etiology of lymphadenopathy [18].

8.4   Dengue-Induced Splenomegaly

Normal spleen weighs around 50–250 g depending on patient's health. Splenomegaly is referred to enlargement of the spleen and measured by estimating the size or weight of the organ. The physiology of the spleen is diversified with active roles in hematopoiesis and immunosurveillance [19]. The histopathological reports of dengue-associated death cases suggest that DENV has potential to target both the spleen and lymph nodes [2]. There are numerous reports indicating the several lesions in the splenic tissues, such as splenic rupture and bleeding, interstitial edema, and vascular congestion [7, 20].

8.4.1   Pathogenesis of Dengue-Induced Splenomegaly

The pathophysiology of splenomegaly during DVI might be attributed to the replication of DENV in the spleen. Moreover, macrophages with replicating dengue virus have been identified morphologically in the affected spleen [21].

8.4.2   Clinical Manifestations of Dengue-Induced Splenomegaly

Patients with splenomegaly present with diverse spectrum of clinical manifestations. Since majority of the diseases of spleen are of secondary nature, a patient presenting with splenomegaly may have a wide pool of signs, symptoms, and test results. These clinical manifestations are also common in various benign or self-limiting and infective or malignant diseases. Clinicians must take cautions and should adopt a systematic approach to identify underlying serious disease while minimizing unnecessary investigations and patient's anxiety [22]. A symptomatic splenomegaly has been reported in literature, and physician's expertise in identification of the condition is of paramount importance [23].

8.4.3   Diagnosis of Dengue-Induced Splenomegaly

Splenomegaly can be identified with physical examination. Cautions must be carried out because spleen size does not always relate to splenic functions and palpable spleens are not always abnormal. The physical examination should include palpation with the patient in the supine and right lateral decubitus position, with knees up and hips flexed [22]. Histopathological analysis of the spleen shows severe parenchymal and circulatory dysfunctions. A comparative analysis of spleen between dengue fatal cases and non-dengue cases demonstrated that spleen of non-dengue patients shows normal regular morphology with normal splenocytes and well-defined demarcation of white and red pulp. On the other hand, prominent parenchymal lesions with remarkable atrophy of lymphoid follicles, disruption of the structural pattern, and destruction of germinal centers have been observed in dengue patients. Quantitative analysis of lymphoid follicle areas in dengue patients may reveal reduced number of follicles in the white pulp region. In addition, vacuolization around degenerated splenocytes and loss of sinusoidal endothelium might be during analysis of semi- and ultrathin sections of the spleen [21].

8.4.4 Management of Splenomegaly

Treatment of underlying primary disorder causing splenomegaly is mainstay of patient's management and can result in regression of hypersplenism without any surgical intervention. However, severe hypersplenism or significantly enlarged spleens can be subjected to splenectomy [24]. However, for patients with hematologic disorders, radiotherapy in low doses has been used as palliative care for the management of splenomegaly [25].

8.5 Dengue-Induced Lymph Node Infarction

Lymph nodes are an important component of the immune system and play a crucial role in both innate and adaptive immune responses. As lymph crosses the nodal parenchyma, antigens are brought in contact with the effector cells of the adaptive immune system resulting in a series of immune processes. These immune responses facilitate the recognition and ultimately neutralization of pathogens and antigens. Blood enters the lymph node through hilar arterioles and exits via venules. Blood circulates through specialized vascular segments (high-endothelial venules) within the lymph node. Lymph nodes are a component of secondary lymphoid system. This system is comprised of the spleen and mucosa-associated lymphoid tissue. Bone marrow and thymus (the sites of B-cell and T-cell production) are primary lymphoid organs [26, 27].

Lymph node infarction is defined as confluent coagulative necrosis of all or a proportion of the lymph node parenchyma, presumably as a result of ischemia. The majority of lymph node infarction cases are associated with past or future malignancy (neoplastic). The nonmalignant causes of lymph node infarction include venous thrombosis, arterial occlusion in vasculitis (polyarteritis nodosa), cholesterol atheromatous emboli, fine-needle aspiration, infectious mononucleosis, post-mediastinoscopy, mononeuritis multiplex, heart–lung transplantation, gold injection, parvovirus B19 viral infection, and intestinal volvulus [28–30].

There are few reports of lymph node infarction in literature as lymph nodes are well vascularized and have well-developed anastomosis of blood vessels [31]. The presence of lymph node infarction in DVI is extremely rare, and there is only one reported case. In this case, laboratory-confirmed DVI patient has lymph node infarction in association with disseminated intravascular coagulation (DIC). Hypothetical analysis demonstrated that lymph node infarction occurred before the DIC became clinically evident. During the case management, the initial treatment with ceftriaxone resulted in shock, cyanosis, and acute kidney injury. However, patient responded and recovered with the administration of steroids, inotropes, and antibiotics including amoxicillin and ceftazidime [32].

All neoplastic and nonneoplastic causes of lymph node infarction as discussed earlier should be ruled at first. Other conditions precipitating node infarction may include necrotizing mucocutaneous lymph node syndrome, lymphadenitis (Kikuchi's lymphadenitis), and necrotizing granulomatous inflammation. Histopathological and microscopic evaluations are considered as promising diagnostic tools for node infarction. Histologically, the lymph node parenchyma shows extensive coagulative necrosis in which pyknotic or completely necrotic cells are present [31]. Since malignant lymphoma is the most common cause of spontaneous lymph node infarction, pathologists should consider the propensity of malignant lymphoma if there is an evidence of completely infarcted lymph nodes [29]. Further investigations should be done to visualize subcapsular tissue for any sign of malignancy. This is usually done by taking out multiple sections of the lymph node from the deeper layer. Immunohistochemistry is carried out on the infarcted lymph node sections to rule out the underlying pathology. The suitability of necrotic tissue for immunohistochemical study is still contradictory [33, 34]. Both infarcted and non-infarcted lymph node in the only reported case did not demonstrate any predisposing condition. However, the examination of parahilar vessels revealed thrombotic occlusion, which might be only a contributor factor of infarction in this case [32].

8.6 Clinical Implications for Healthcare Professionals

Lymphoreticular involvements in dengue infection are extremely rare. However, they may occur any time during the clinical course of infection. Since lymphoreticular complications are fatal, awareness of these intricacies among physicians, particularly in dengue endemic areas, is of utmost importance. A case of splenic rupture can be misdiagnosed with shock syndrome among patients with DSS. For splenic rupture, splenectomy can be curative, but it must be considered for severe patients only. Malignant lymphoma, being the most common cause of lymph node infarction, should be ruled out earliest through immunohistochemistry. The risk of development of malignant lymphoma is high within the 2 years of infarction; thereby, patients should be followed up at least for high-risk period.

References

1. Gulati S, Maheshwari A. Atypical manifestations of dengue. Tropical Med Int Health. 2007;12(9):1087–95.
2. Bhamarapravati N, Tuchinda P, Boonyapaknavik V. Pathology of Thailand haemorrhagic fever: a study of 100 autopsy cases. Ann Trop Med Parasitol. 1967;61(4):500–10.
3. Aung-Khin M, Ma-Ma K. Changes in the tissues of the immune system in dengue haemorrhagic fever. J Trop Med Hyg. 1975;78(12):256–61.

4. Mebius RE, Kraal G. Structure and function of the spleen. Nat Rev Immunol. 2005;5(8):606.
5. Weaver H, Kumar V, Spencer K, Maatouk M, Malik S. Spontaneous splenic rupture: a rare life-threatening condition; Diagnosed early and managed successfully. Am J Case Rep. 2013;14:13.
6. Gedik E, Girgin S, Aldemir M, Keles C, Tuncer MC, Aktas A. Non-traumatic splenic rupture: report of seven cases and review of the literature. World J Gastroenterol. 2008;14(43):6711.
7. Bhaskar E, Moorthy S. Spontaneous splenic rupture in dengue fever with non-fatal outcome in an adult. J Infect Dev Ctries. 2012;6(04):369–72.
8. Mukhopadhyay M, Chatterjee N, Maity P, Patar K. Spontaneous splenic rupture: a rare presentation of dengue fever. Indian J Crit Care Med. 2014;18(2):110.
9. Silva W, Gunasekera M. Spontaneous splenic rupture during the recovery phase of dengue fever. BMC Res Notes. 2015;8(1):286.
10. de Souza LJ, de Azevedo J, Kohler LIA, de Freitas Barros L, Lima MA, Silva EM, et al. Evidence of dengue virus replication in a non-traumatic spleen rupture case. Arch Virol. 2017;162(11):3535–9.
11. Gopie P, Teelucksingh S, Naraynsingh V. Splenic rupture mimicking dengue shock syndrome. Trop Gastroenterol. 2012;33(2):154–5.
12. Aubrey-Bassler FK, Sowers N. 613 cases of splenic rupture without risk factors or previously diagnosed disease: a systematic review. BMC Emerg Med. 2012;12(1):11.
13. Vick LR, Islam S. Recombinant factor VIIa as an adjunct in nonoperative management of solid organ injuries in children. J Pediatr Surg. 2008;43(1):195–9.
14. Giagounidis A, Burk M, Meckenstock G, Koch A, Schneider W. Pathologic rupture of the spleen in hematologic malignancies: two additional cases. Ann Hematol. 1996;73(6):297–302.
15. Pothapregada S, Kamalakannan B, Thulasingam M. Clinical profile of atypical manifestations of dengue fever. Indian J Pediatr. 2016;83(6):493–9.
16. Sreenivasulu T, Jahnavi K. A study of clinical profile of patients with Dengue fever at a tertiary care hospital. Int J Adv Med. 2018;5(1):202–6.
17. Blackley S, Kou Z, Chen H, Quinn M, Rose RC, Schlesinger JJ, et al. Primary human splenic macrophages, but not T or B cells, are the principal target cells for dengue virus infection in vitro. J Virol. 2007;81(24):13325–34.
18. Nield LS, Kamat D. Lymphadenopathy in children: when and how to evaluate. Clin Pediatr. 2004;43(1):25–33.
19. Papenfuss TL, Cesta MF. Spleen. Immunopathology in toxicology and drug development. Cham: Springer; 2017. p. 37–57.
20. Basílio-de-Oliveira C, Aguiar G, Baldanza M, Barth O, Eyer-Silva W, Paes M. Pathologic study of a fatal case of dengue-3 virus infection in Rio de Janeiro, Brazil. Braz J Infect Dis. 2005;9(4):341–7.
21. Póvoa TF, Alves AM, Oliveira CA, Nuovo GJ, Chagas VL, Paes MV. The pathology of severe dengue in multiple organs of human fatal cases: histopathology, ultrastructure and virus replication. PLoS One. 2014;9(4):e83386.
22. Pozo AL, Godfrey EM, Bowles KM. Splenomegaly: investigation, diagnosis and management. Blood Rev. 2009;23(3):105–11.
23. Hesdorffer C, Macfarlane B, Sandler M, Grant S, Ziady F. True idiopathic splenomegaly-a distinct clinical entity. Eur J Haematol. 1986;37(4):310–5.
24. Subhasis RC, Rajiv C, Kumar SA, Kumar AV, Kumar PA. Surgical treatment of massive splenomegaly and severe hypersplenism secondary to extrahepatic portal venous obstruction in children. Surg Today. 2007;37(1):19–23.
25. Lavrenkov K, Krepel-Volsky S, Levi I, Ariad S. Low dose palliative radiotherapy for splenomegaly in hematologic disorders. Leuk Lymphoma. 2012;53(3):430–4.
26. Swartz MA. The physiology of the lymphatic system. Adv Drug Deliv Rev. 2001;50(1-2):3–20.
27. Willard-Mack CL. Normal structure, function, and histology of lymph nodes. Toxicol Pathol. 2006;34(5):409–24.
28. Pinto RGW, Couto F, Mandreker S. Infarction after fine needle aspiration. Acta Cytol. 1996;40(4):739–41.

29. Roberts C, Batstone P, Goodlad J. Lymphadenopathy and lymph node infarction as a result of gold injections. J Clin Pathol. 2001;54(7):562–4.
30. Srujana S, Srivani N, Krishna L, Kumar OS, Quadri SS. A rare case of lymph node infarction. Int Surg J. 2016;2(1):98–101.
31. Arno J. Atlas of lymph node pathology. New York: Springer Science & Business Media; 2012.
32. Rao IS, Loya AC, Ratnakar K, Srinivasan V. Lymph node infarction—a rare complication associated with disseminated intra vascular coagulation in a case of dengue fever. BMC Clin Pathol. 2005;5(1):11.
33. Strauchen JA, Miller LK. Lymph node infarction: an immunohistochemical study of 11 cases. Arch Pathol Lab Med. 2003;127(1):60–3.
34. Norton AJ, Ramsay AD, Isaacson PG. Antigen preservation in infarcted lymphoid tissue. A novel approach to the infarcted lymph node using monoclonal antibodies effective in routinely processed tissues. Am J Surg Pathol. 1988;12(10):759–67.

Dengue-Induced Ocular Complications

9

9.1 Ocular Involvements in Dengue Infection

The occurrence of ocular involvements during the course of dengue virus infection (DVI) has been increasing. The prevalence of dengue-associated ocular complications has been estimated up to 40% [1, 2]. Ocular diseases could present as part of the vascular and hemorrhagic phenomena caused by DVI. Dengue eye disease can be either unilateral or bilateral. The appearance of ocular symptoms following the onset of the DVI takes around 2–5 months following the onset of fever. However, most of the ocular symptoms have been observed within 24 h of the nadir of thrombocytopenia (~7 days after the onset of fever) [1]. Currently the mechanisms underlying the pathogenesis of dengue-associated ophthalmic complications are not precisely clear; however, many studies have alluded to the propensity of immune-mediated process as potential contributor of ocular intricacies [1, 3, 4]. There is a wide spectrum of dengue-associated ophthalmic complications including retinal vasculitis, retinal edema, anterior uveitis, optic neuritis, ischemic optic neuropathy, retinal pigment epithelial disturbance, exudative retinal detachment, and branch retinal artery occlusion.

9.2 Predictors of Dengue-Related Eye Disease

Several predisposing factors contribute to the development of ocular complications during the course of DVI. Dengue maculopathy has been reported to be serotype specific. Existing literature indicate that dengue virus serotype 1 (DENV-1) epidemic is associated with dengue-induced eye diseases, while there is no such association with DENV-2 epidemic [5]. However, there is a need of further investigations to draw firm conclusion on the relationship of DENV serotype and ocular pathogenesis in DVI. Other significant contributors of ocular symptoms are hypoalbuminemia and leukopenia. Hypoalbuminemia may increase the vascular permeability, while leukopenia could predispose to opportunistic infection of the ocular tissues, resulting in various eye pathologies [6].

© Springer Nature Singapore Pte Ltd. 2021
T. H. Mallhi et al., *Expanded Dengue Syndrome*,
https://doi.org/10.1007/978-981-15-7337-8_9

9.3   Common Ocular Symptoms in Dengue Infection

Recent evidences from the available literature indicate that ophthalmic manifestations in dengue infection are uncommon but not rare. The rate of maculopathy is observed as 10% in a case series conducted among hospitalized DVI cases [4]. The chief ocular complaints in dengue patients are eye strain (30%), retroocular pain (20%), blurred vision (10%), foreign body sensation (3%), diplopia (3%), photopsia (2%), and floaters (1%) [6]. Blurred vision (60%) and central scotomata (30%) are primary ophthalmic manifestations among patients with established ocular pathology associated with DVI. One third of the dengue patients have bilateral involvement and visual acuity ranging from 20/20 to counting fingers (CF), with a median of 20/40 [7].

Blurred vision with visual acuity ranging from 6.0/7.5 to CF has been experienced by many dengue patients [8]. However, patients with dengue-related maculopathy may present with vision worse than LogMAR 0.15 [4]. Blurred vision accounts approximately half of the dengue-related maculopathies [1]. It has been observed cystoid macular edema is associated with poorer visual acuity. The amount of macular edema correlates with the degree of visual loss and prognosis [3].

Central scotoma is the second most common ocular manifestations related to the dengue infection. It occurs in association with blurring of vision in most of the cases [8]. The areas of scotoma correspond to the areas of edema and hemorrhage in the macula [9]. Ocular pain is another disturbing complaint experienced by DVI patients. Available data described the location of pain as retrobulbar or diffused. It must be noted that retrobulbar pain is also primarily associated with the other complications including retinopathy sparing the macula, subconjunctival hemorrhage, retinal hemorrhages, and stellar neuroretinitis [10].

9.4   Spectrum of Dengue-Induced Ophthalmic Complications

Since the structure of eye is stratified into anterior and posterior segments, clinical features of dengue-related eye disease can be morphologically categorized as described in Table 9.1.

9.4.1   Dengue-Induced Anterior Segment Complications

9.4.1.1 Subconjunctival Hemorrhage
Unilateral or bilateral subconjunctival hemorrhage is a common finding in dengue fever. Regardless of the platelet count, its reported incidence ranges from 8 to 60 [2]. Dengue-induced subconjunctival hemorrhage has also been reported among dengue patients under critical care in ICU [12]. Petechial hemorrhages are commonly observed hemorrhagic type among dengue patients. The relationship of

Table 9.1 Ocular complications during dengue infection

Complications of anterior segment of the eye
Subconjunctival hemorrhage
Anterior uveitis
Intermediate uveitis
Shallow anterior chamber
Ciliary congestion
Keratitis
Corneal erosion
Acute angle closure
Complications of posterior segment of the eye
Maculopathy
Macular edema
Vitreous hemorrhage
Vascular occlusions (vein occlusions)
Arterial occlusion of the superotemporal macular branch
Retinal hemorrhages
Posterior uveitis
Foveolitis
Serous retinal detachment
Neuro-ophthalmic disorders
Optic neuritis
Cranial nerve palsies
Neuromyelitis optica
Miscellaneous ophthalmic complications
Panophthalmitis
Periorbital ecchymosis

Sources: Table is self-constructed and data is extracted from references [10, 11]

platelet count and subconjunctival hemorrhage is not well established as this complication has been observed in patients with platelet counts <50,000/μL and even in patients having thrombocytopenia of 13,000–40,000/μL [2, 12].

9.4.1.2 Anterior Uveitis

Uveitis rarely manifests during the course of DVI. However, anterior uveitis counts 7.7% of ocular symptoms in dengue infection. However, its incidence in patients with concurrent maculopathy is reported as 17%. Both unilateral and bilateral involvements have been observed in DVI. In addition to the uveitis of anterior chamber, panuveitis can occur among dengue patients. Its clinical diagnosis is primarily based on the ophthalmic symptoms including photophobia and redness and signs of keratic precipitates, perilimbal injection, and anterior chamber cells [1, 13–15]. It must be noted that anterior uveitis usually occurs after 3–5 months following DVI. It is suggested that the late onset of uveitis on the context of full systemic recovery indicates immunologic mechanisms in the pathogenesis of uveitis [15].

9.4.1.3 Intermediate Uveitis

The prevalence of intermediate uveitis ranges from 3.2 to 12.3% of dengue-associated ocular symptoms [3, 16]. Several epidemiological studies have reported occurrence of vitritis in 31% and concurrent appearance of both anterior and intermediate uveitis in 11% patients with dengue maculopathy [15].

9.4.1.4 Other Anterior Chamber Complications of Dengue Infection

Corneal pathology is quite rare during the course of dengue infection and only explains in separate case reports. Patients with DVI are reported to have bilateral punctate lower corneal erosions during the infection course [17]. The other corneal involvements include peripheral hypopyon corneal ulcer in severe cases (DSS), retrobulbar hemorrhage complicated by corneal perforation, and endophthalmitis [12, 18].

Shallow anterior chambers have also been described through separate case reports [19–21]. Out of the five eyes examined in these reports, acute angle closure was diagnosed in three cases. Moreover, bilateral involvement is also observed in one patient [20, 21]. Among patients with bilateral choroidal effusions, the intraocular pressure remains within the normal range. However, pressure may elevate with the occurrence of angle closure glaucoma during infection [19, 20]. The relationship between shallow anterior chamber and DVI is needed to be determined. It is unclear from the findings of available case reports if these complications are incidental or related to the DVI.

There is also a report describing incidence of ciliary congestion along with uveitis in patient with DVI [15].

9.4.2   Dengue-Induced Posterior Segment Complications

9.4.2.1 Maculopathy

Dengue maculopathy is the most studied ophthalmic complication of DVI with estimated prevalence of about 10% [4]. The occurrence of maculopathy is also associated with DENV serotype. Existing data indicate no relationship of maculopathy with DENV-2 [9]. The clinical manifestations of maculopathy can be observed between 6 and 7 days after onset of fever. However, some patients also experience the symptoms even after 30 days of infection [1]. Visual symptoms can occur in patients hospitalized with dengue maculopathy [4]. The primary visual complaints associated with dengue maculopathy are blurred vision, scotomata, and floaters. Less common symptoms include micropsia and metamorphopsia [3, 16]. Dengue maculopathy may associate with initial mean best-corrected visual acuity (BCVA) ranging from 20/40 to 20/45. Initial BCVA worse than 20/25 and 20/40 has been observed among dengue cases at the time of hospital presentation. Poorer BCVA has been seen in patients with macular edema and foveolitis, which is assumed to be correlated with the severity of macular edema. Bilateral, but asymmetric, involvement has been observed in patients during the course of DVI [1, 3]. Existing data indicate the incidences of macular edema and macular hemorrhage as of 77 and

69%, respectively, with arteriolar sheathing, cotton wool spots, perifoveal telangiectasia, and microaneurysms [3, 8]. Dengue-related maculopathy-induced hemorrhages can be in the form of flame-shaped hemorrhages, dot, or blot. Most of these hemorrhages are intraretinal [1].

It has been suggested that the incidence of maculopathy is associated with the severity of systemic disease. The overall incidence of ocular complications in DVI patients is approximately 8% [15], and dengue maculopathy may occur in up to 10% hospitalized patients with DVI [4]. The prevalence of dengue maculopathy may increase up to 40% in severe patients (DHF and DSS) requiring admission to intensive care unit (ICU) [12].

9.4.2.2 Macular Edema

Macular edema is the most frequent presentation of dengue-related maculopathy [3, 8, 16]. Macular edema can be categorized based on appearance on optical coherence tomography (OCT). The following are the three patterns of macular edema on OCT [3]:

- Type 1 (diffuse edema)
- Type 2 (cystoid edema)
- Type 3 (cystic foveolitis)

Dengue-induced macular edema has primarily been explained through isolated case reports [22, 23]. Macular edema frequently presents among symptomatic patients. Available literature indicates that DVI patients with ocular complications may have an extensive panretinal vasculitis with exudative retinal detachment in about 20% cases [16]. Macular hemorrhage is another most frequent presentation of dengue maculopathy. Fundoscopic examination shows scattered blot and flame hemorrhages, as described above [24]. It is interesting to note that macular hemorrhage also corresponds to the areas of scotomata [8].

9.4.2.3 Retinal Hemorrhage

Retinal hemorrhage during the course of DVI is an independent contributor to the visual symptoms. Dengue-associated retinal hemorrhage possesses bilateral involvement and may present with decreased visual acuity and metamorphopsia. Blot hemorrhages within the vascular arcades can also occur as unifying findings. All the hemorrhages affecting the macula result in visual manifestations [25]. A triad of blurred vision, photopsia, and floaters is strongly associated with retinal hemorrhages. All these three symptoms have 100% positive predictive value for the presence of retinal hemorrhages which may or may not affect the macula [6].

9.4.2.4 Foveolitis

Foveolitis is a pathological condition of the fovea which is characterized by well-defined yellowish subretinal lesions in the macula along with retinal striae radiating around the fovea. These lesions correspond to disruption of the outer neurosensory retina and the inner segment/outer segment (IS/OS) junction. Simply it refers to the yellow–orange lesion at the fovea of patients with dengue maculopathy, which corresponds to a disruption of the outer neurosensory retina in OCT [14]. Before the term foveolitis was coined, similar complications are termed as yellow subretinal dots across the published literature [1, 4]. Foveolitis along with maculopathy has been observed in 28–33.7% DVI cases [1, 3]. Bilateral foveolitis can occur which may present with concurrent findings of superior temporal branch vein occlusion and macula edema. Symptoms can be observed from 5 to 9 days following onset of fever. Dengue-associated foveolitis is sometimes accompanied by BCVA ranging from 20/25 to CF. The worse BCVA in dengue patients at presentation is reported to be associated with larger lesions, central scotomata, and hyperfluorescence at the fovea on fundus fluorescein angiography (FFA). However, central scotoma has been seen in up to 100% of patients with dengue-related foveolitis [3, 14].

9.4.2.5 Vascular Occlusions
Vascular occlusions are less frequent ocular complications of DVI. Both venous and arterial occlusions have been observed during the course of dengue infection and are described in isolated case reports [14, 23, 24, 26]. Most of these reports discuss cases of venous occlusions, and only one case of branch retinal artery occlusion is reported in the literature [26]. It has been observed that vascular occlusions occur independently without any association with other ophthalmic manifestations of DVI. Patient who was presented with arterial occlusion in the literature had 2 weeks history of inferior nasal field deficit corresponding to the fundus signs of retinal whitening in the superotemporal quadrant of the macula, with attenuation and sclerosis of the macular division of the superotemporal branch retinal artery [26]. On the other hand, patients with branch vein occlusion may present with concurrent features of retinal vasculitis, foveolitis, and bilateral macular edema [14]. The presence of vasculitic vein occlusion in these cases suggests an inflammatory mechanism.

9.4.2.6 Optic Neuropathy
The common presentations of dengue-related optic neuropathy include disc hemorrhages, optic disc swelling, and hyperemia. Optic disc swelling and hyperemia are less common presentations among patients with dengue-related maculopathy which account 14% and 11%, respectively. It must be noted that optic disc swelling may progress to optic atrophy with a visual acuity of no light perception [27]. Optic neuropathy is relatively uncommon compared to other dengue-related ocular signs [1].

9.4.2.7 Posterior Uveitis and Panuveitis
Posterior uveitis is a relatively common intricacy of DVI. Its spectrum of manifestations revolves around retinitis, neuroretinitis, and chorioretinitis. Retinal and panretinal vasculitis with exudative retinal detachment and posterior vitreous cells have been reported during the course of dengue infection [16]. Both focal and multifocal chorioretinitis may occur and more often associates with macular pathology [28].

Dengue patients with bilateral multifocal retinochoroiditis sometimes appear with concurrent retinal hemorrhages and bilateral retinal vasculitis [29]. Dry atrophic perifoveal pigmentary changes may develop after the initial episode of inflammatory chorioretinitis [28]. These findings are also described as nummular-shaped pigmented scars [29]. Dengue infection may also present with bilateral stellar neuroretinitis, and there is only one case report describing bilateral stellar neuroretinitis in Brazilian patients who also had bilateral vitritis, papillitis, macular star exudates, and areas of serous retinal detachment [30].

Unilateral panophthalmitis during dengue infection has been documented in only two children in the literature. In one case panophthalmitis was attributed to the direct injury by the DENV [21]. In second patient, panophthalmitis and orbital cellulitis was thought to be a result of occult maxillary sinusitis and DVI [31].

9.5 Pathogenesis of Dengue-Induced Ophthalmic Complications

Dengue-related eye disease has been postulated to be caused by various factors associated with pathogenesis. These include viral virulence, host susceptibility, DENV serotypes, geographic factors, mutations, and the wide range of clinical manifestations during the course of disease. Multifactorial pathophysiological mechanisms are also involved in the pathogenesis of dengue-associated ophthalmic complications. Thrombocytopenia and immune-mediated mechanisms indirectly contribute towards dengue eye disease by inducing the ocular hemorrhage [11].

The association of thrombocytopenia with ocular hemorrhages has been vigorously tested in several studies and found as a significant contributor of eye complications during the course of DVI [2]. However, immune pathogenesis has also been evidenced by the natural history of dengue ophthalmic disease. It must be noted that majority of ocular manifestations occur at the nadir of thrombocytopenia. Since systemic immunologic response increases after 7 days of onset of fever, the propensity of ocular complications is high during this period [16]. The association between low complement C3 and C4 levels and maculopathy has been documented in the literature [4]. Patients who have no systemic illnesses may also present with uveitis of no other detectable cause even after 3–5 months of DVI [15]. Moreover, improvement in ocular manifestations following the high-dose steroidal therapy suggests the involvement of immune mechanisms. All these findings strongly support immunological pathogenesis of dengue eye disease.

A case series conducted on severe dengue cases having maculopathy shows that intravenous immunoglobulin therapy causes persistent low C4 levels among patients [1]. Similar results have been noticed by Chang et al. that patients who developed retinal vasculitis, vitreous hemorrhage, and maculopathy have isolated low C4 levels. These findings postulate that a low C4 level may predispose to immune complex formation when triggered by dengue viremia [5]. However, the association of persistently low C4 levels with disease severity is still not clear.

9.6   Diagnosis of Spectrum of Dengue-Induced Ophthalmic Complications

Several ocular investigations have been suggested to assess the ophthalmic complications during DVI. Table 9.2 provides the list of investigations which can be used to facilitate the diagnostic workup [1, 10, 11].

Table 9.2 Investigational methods used to assess or diagnose dengue-induced ophthalmic complications

Investigational method	Use
Amsler charting	This method is used to map out visual field changes and scotomata in dengue-related maculopathy
Fundus fluorescein angiography (FFA)	This test is used to map out visual field, mainly vascular occlusion or leakage, and used to aid the diagnosis of vein occlusions and vasculitis
Optical coherence tomography (OCT)	OCT is used to evaluate the retinal thickness and morphology
Neuroimaging	Magnetic resonance imaging (MRI) has been used infrequently in a few specific situations. MRI has demonstrated enhancement of the optic nerve sheath complex in retrobulbar optic neuritis and is also used to confirm the diagnosis of panophthalmitis in one patient after initial investigation with ultrasound. MRI of the brain and spinal cord is also used in the diagnosis of NMO. Computed tomography scans were used to diagnose orbital hematoma as well as a concurrent subarachnoid hemorrhage
Automated Humphrey visual field analysis (HVF)	This method is used to map out visual field changes and scotomata
Indocyanine green angiography (ICG)	ICG is used to evaluate visual field, occlusions, and leaking. ICG is a better diagnostic method for foveolitis than FFA
Electrophysiological testing	Various electrophysiologic modalities used include pattern electroretinogram (Perg), full fundus electroretinogram (ffERG), multifocal electroretinogram (mfERG), and visual evoked potentials (VEPs). Electrophysiology tests were less commonly performed
Microperimetry	Serial microperimetry is considered a preferred method to monitor dengue-related maculopathy with central scotomata. Microperimetry is more sensitive and is able to monitor a reduction in the size of scotomata, which is not detectable on Goldmann perimetry
Fundus autofluorescence	This test is used to evaluate a patient with maculopathy
Infrared fundus photography	This method is rarely used. It can be utilized to document maculopathy

Sources: This table is self-constructed. Data is extracted from references [1, 10, 11]

9.7 Management of Dengue-Induced Ophthalmic Complications

Most of the cases with dengue eye disease are treated conservatively. However, platelet transfusion might be required in patients with thrombocytopenia. Currently, there is no established therapy for dengue maculopathy. Moreover, lack of randomized controlled trials further underscore the attention of healthcare researchers towards this least appreciated area. Since available studies conducted on the treatment of dengue maculopathy lack control group for comparison, it is not possible to draw a firm conclusion or comment on the benefits of the treatment. Most of these studies are case series and provide broad information on the clinical presentation of the disease, active surveillance, and corticosteroid therapy as treatment modalities among cases. Based on the findings of these studies, it is not clear evidence that whether immunosuppressive therapy improves the prognosis or hastens the clinical recovery among patients with dengue maculopathy [13].

Most of the dengue-related eye diseases are self-limited and resolve spontaneously over time. Existing literature have demonstrated spontaneous recovery for retinal or macular hemorrhages, foveolitis, subconjunctival hemorrhages, posterior uveitis, and optic neuritis. Some conditions like subconjunctival hemorrhages have been reported to be resolved within 6–14 days [2]. However, recovery time varies across the studies ranging from 3 to 14 days [8, 14, 25, 27, 29]. However, few studies have demonstrated impaired color vision and paracentral scotoma even after the 10 months of treatment [27]. There is dire need of active surveillance for dengue eye disease recovery and resolution to establish treatment guidelines and to define the duration of treatment according to patient's condition.

9.7.1 Corticosteroids

Corticosteroids are considered mainstay of therapy for dengue-related ocular complications. Steroids provide substantial improvements in persistently symptomatic patients or those who have poor vision due to dengue eye disease. Both topical and systematic administrations of steroids are used depending on the ophthalmic involvement. Topical prednisolone 1% is used for patients with dengue-related uveitis [15, 16]. Patients who do not respond to topical steroids can be considered for oral prednisolone. Patients with visual acuity worse than 6/60 and those who do not respond to the initial treatment strategies (i.e. oral prednisolone) can be managed with intravenous methylprednisolone. Periocular methylprednisolone injections can also be used for unilateral disease [1]. Available literature indicates that intravenous methylprednisolone can be used with intravenous immunoglobulin for patients having dengue-related maculopathy and visual acuity of 6/120 or worse [14].

Table 9.3 Treatment strategies for dengue maculopathy

Eye condition	Strategies
Patients who are symptomatic, have a BCVA of 20/40 or worse in the affected eye, and/or have subjectively persistent or progressive deterioration of vision	Systemic steroids (follow-up time for patients treated with systemic corticosteroids ranged from 1 to 15 weeks)
Patients with bilateral disease	Oral prednisolone (1 mg/kg tapered according to ocular response or development of adverse reactions)
If BCVA are severely depressed (20/200 or worse) and/or without improvement after 3 days of initial oral corticosteroid treatment	IV methylprednisolone 1 g/day for 3 days, followed by oral prednisolone
If no improvement is noted after 3 days of IV methylprednisolone	Intravenous immunoglobulin (IVIG) (400 mg/kg for 5 days)

Sources: Table is self-constructed and information is extracted from reference [1]

Subconjunctival dexamethasone, sub-Tenon's triamcinolone [15], and intravitreal triamcinolone acetonide [1, 13] are some other forms of local corticosteroids used for the management of dengue-associated ophthalmic complications. However, dengue patients who develop uveitis, maculopathy, NMO, or optic neuritis may get benefits with systemic steroidal therapy [11].

Available literature provides several strategies to manage dengue maculopathy. These strategies are described in Table 9.3 [1]. It has been noted that steroidal treatment shows promising benefits among patients with intraretinal choroidal or vascular leakage, with foveal swelling, and with evidence of active ocular inflammation. On the other hand, patients having vaso-occlusive disease are associated with residual scotomata even with the optimum therapy [1].

Systemic steroids have also demonstrated promising activity against extensive panretinal vasculitis, exudative retinal detachment, and optic neuritis [16, 27]. The treatment of ophthalmic complications by both systemic and oral steroids carries favorable visual outcome among dengue patients.

9.7.2   Intravenous Immunoglobulin (IVIG)

Patients who do not respond to systemic corticosteroid therapy can be treated with IVIG (0.4 g/kg/day for 3 days). Vision improvement after the 15 days of initiation of IVIG has been documented in the literature [5]. Visual outcomes following intravenous immunoglobulin treatment are generally favorable.

9.7.3   Other Interventions for Dengue Eye Diseases

Several other interventions have been tested in dengue eye disease. Pars plana vitrectomy can be used for vitreous hemorrhage. For acute angle closure, peripheral iridotomy and ocular hypotensive agents have been proved to provide promising results. Retinal hypoperfusion can be treated with panretinal photocoagulation. Preretinal hemorrhage is a useful measure to prevent neovascularization [8, 16].

9.8   Prognosis of Dengue Eye Disease

The prognosis of dengue eye disease depends on the nature and severity of the eye involvement. Patients with ocular involvements may have spontaneous resolution of symptoms or sometimes may lead to blindness even during the treatment. Patients may experience color vision impairment and persistent paracentral scotoma even after several months of clinical resolution. This scotoma is reflected as an area of decreased sensitivity through HVF, microperimetry, and Amsler grid. Dengue patients having foveal inflammation, either clinically or on OCT, and ischemia on FFA show poorer outcomes. However, the prognosis for central visual acuity is quite better, and sometimes more than 80% of patients achieve a final BCVA of 20/40 or more [16]. The best prognosis has been seen in type I diffuse retinal thickness where mean BCVA at 2 years is reported as 20/25 and 69.7% resolution of scotomata. The mean BCVA at 2 years of 20/25 has been recorded in type II cystoid macular edema with 43.8% resolution of scotomata. The mean BCVA at 2 years is 20/25 in type III foveolitis, but scotomata may persist despite clinical and anatomical resolution [3].

References

1. Bacsal KE, Chee S-P, Cheng C-L, Flores JVP. Dengue-associated maculopathy. Arch Ophthalmol. 2007;125(4):501–10.
2. Kapoor HK, Bhai S, John M, Xavier J. Ocular manifestations of dengue fever in an East Indian epidemic. Can J Ophthalmol. 2006;41(6):741–6.
3. Teoh S, Chee C, Laude A, Goh K, Barkham T, Ang B, et al. Optical coherence tomography patterns as predictors of visual outcome in dengue-related maculopathy. Retina. 2010;30(3):390–8.
4. Su DH-W, Bacsal K, Chee S-P, Flores JVP, Lim W-K, Cheng BC-L, et al. Prevalence of dengue maculopathy in patients hospitalized for dengue fever. Ophthalmology. 2007;114(9):1743–7.e4.
5. Chang P, Cheng C, Asok K, Fong K, Chee S, Tan C. Visual disturbances in dengue fever: an answer at last. Singap Med J. 2007;48(3):71–3.
6. Seet RC, Quek AM, Lim EC. Symptoms and risk factors of ocular complications following dengue infection. J Clin Virol. 2007;38(2):101–5.
7. Tan MH, Tan P, Wong E, Chen FK. Structure and function correlation in a patient with dengue-associated maculopathy. Clin Exp Ophthalmol. 2014;42(5):504.
8. Chan DP, Teoh SC, Tan CS, Nah GK, Rajagopalan R, Prabhakaragupta MK, et al. Ophthalmic complications of dengue. Emerg Infect Dis. 2006;12(2):285.
9. Chee E, Sims JL, Jap A, Tan BH, Oh H, Chee S-P. Comparison of prevalence of dengue maculopathy during two epidemics with differing predominant serotypes. Am J Ophthalmol. 2009;148(6):910–3.
10. Yip VC-H, Sanjay S, Koh YT. Ophthalmic complications of dengue fever: a systematic review. Ophthalmol Therapy. 2012;1(1):2.
11. Ng AW, Teoh SC. Dengue eye disease. Surv Ophthalmol. 2015;60(2):106–14.
12. Mehta S, Mehta S, Jiandani P. Ocular features of dengue septic shock (DSS). J Assoc Physicians India. 2006;54(5):866.

13. Antlanger M, Shaw SJ, Kurup SK. Presumed dengue-associated immune-mediated uveitis. Can J Ophthalmol. 2011;46(1):92–3.
14. Loh B-K, Bacsal K, Chee S-P, Cheng BC-L, Wong D. Foveolitis associated with dengue fever: a case series. Ophthalmologica. 2008;222(5):317–20.
15. Gupta A, Srinivasan R, Setia S, Soundravally R, Pandian D. Uveitis following dengue fever. Eye. 2009;23(4):873.
16. Teoh CBS, Chan DP, Nath GKM, Rajagopalan R, Laude A, Ang BSP, et al. A re-look at ocular complications in dengue fever and dengue haemorrhagic fever. Dengue Bulletin. 2006;30:184–90.
17. Chhavi N, Venkatesh C, Soundararajan P, Gunasekaran D. Unusual ocular manifestations of dengue fever in a young girl. Indian J Pediatr. 2013;80(6):1–2.
18. Intizar Hussain F, Afzal F, Doms AS. Ophthalmic manifestation of dengue fever. Off J Peshawar Med Coll. 2012;10(1):93.
19. Cruz-Villegas V, Berrocal AM, Davis JL. Bilateral choroidal effusions associated with dengue fever. Retina. 2003;23(4):576–8.
20. Pierre Filho PTP, Carvalho Filho JP, Pierre ÉTL. Bilateral acute angle closure glaucoma in a patient with dengue fever: case report. Arq Bras Oftalmol. 2008;71(2):265–8.
21. Saranappa SBS, Sowbhagya H. Panophthalmitis in dengue fever. Indian Pediatr. 2012;49(9):760.
22. Habot-Wilner Z, Moisseiev J, Bin H, Rubinovitch B. A returned traveler with dengue fever and visual impairment. Israel Med Assoc J. 2005;7(3):200.
23. Tan C, Teoh S, Chan D, Wong I, Lim T. Dengue retinopathy manifesting with bilateral vasculitis and macular oedema. Eye. 2007;21(6):875.
24. Quek D, Barkham T, Teoh S. Recurrent bilateral dengue maculopathy following sequential infections with two serotypes of dengue virus. Eye. 2009;23(6):1471.
25. Chlebicki MP, Ang B, Barkham T, Laude A. Retinal hemorrhages in 4 patients with dengue fever. Emerg Infect Dis. 2005;11(5):770.
26. Kanungo S, Shukla D, Kim R. Branch retinal artery occlusion secondary to dengue fever. Indian J Ophthalmol. 2008;56(1):73.
27. Sanjay S, Wagle A, Eong KA. Optic neuropathy associated with dengue fever. Eye. 2008;22(5):722.
28. Teoh S, Chan D, Laude A, Chee C, Lim T, Goh K. Dengue chorioretinitis and dengue-related ophthalmic complications. Ocul Immunol Uveitis Found. 2006;9(4):1–19.
29. Tabbara K. Dengue retinochoroiditis. Ann Saudi Med. 2012;32(5):530–3.
30. de Amorim Garcia C, Gomes A, de Oliveira ÁG. Bilateral stellar neuroretinitis in a patient with dengue fever. Eye. 2006;20(12):1382.
31. Molligoda P, Sen P. A case of orbital cellulitis and pan-ophthalmitis in dengue haemorrhagic fever in a child. Sri Lanka J Child Health. 2006;35:38–40.

Dengue-Induced Miscellaneous Complications

10

10.1 Miscellaneous Complications in Dengue Infection

There are several other organ systems infested by the dengue virus (DENV) causing varying complications during the course of dengue viral infection (DVI). The following atypical manifestations are discussed in this chapter:

- Cutaneous complications
- Oral complications
- Intracranial hemorrhage
- Thyroiditis
- Splenial lesion syndrome
- Hemophagocytic lymphohistiocytosis

10.2 Cutaneous Complications in Dengue Infection

Skin is the first site of interaction between DENV and human cells. Female mosquito injects DENV into the skin through mouth parts or proboscis. Virus enters through epidermis into the dermis and reaches to a suitable site where blood can be collected from the capillaries [1]. It is interesting to note that DENV remains detectable in the site of inoculation even after viremia subsided. It indicates that dengue infection remains persistent in the skin even after the resolution of symptoms [2]. Other areas of the skin where clinical manifestations of DVI such as hemorrhage or edema appear are usually not positive for DENV. These lesions are primarily attributed to the systemic inflammatory responses [3]. However, it has been documented in the literature that early appearance of skin-related manifestations such as rash or cutaneous complications are associated with improved disease outcomes among patients [4]. Existing data indicates that onset of DSS activates immune cells in the skin, potentially reflecting the systemic inflammatory response [5].

© Springer Nature Singapore Pte Ltd. 2021
T. H. Mallhi et al., *Expanded Dengue Syndrome*,
https://doi.org/10.1007/978-981-15-7337-8_10

Immune cells of the myeloid lineage are the key targets of DENV at the site of inoculation. These cells include phagocytes, various subsets of dendritic cells (DCs), and monocytes [1]. Animal models have suggested that monocyte-derived DCs are significantly recruited into the skin following DVI [6]. In human skin explants and sites of DENV vaccination, Langerhans cells are also targets of infection as well as CD1c$^+$ and CD14$^+$ dermal DCs [7]. Multiple non-hematopoietic cell types in the skins are also considered as early targets of DENV [8].

Cutaneous signs and symptoms account prominently in the clinical manifestations of DVI. Cutaneous manifestations have been reported in 65% of DVI patients. Of these, morbilliform rash or a confluent erythematous rash with white islands of sparing petechiae is common [4]. Other studies have shown considerable proportion of ankle, leg, and face edema accompanying the classical presentations of DVI [9]. The most uncomfortable dermatological symptom during the course of DVI is pruritus. Morbilliform macules may lead to skin pruritus and swelling of palms or soles [4]. Viral replication primarily in macrophages may contribute to these cutaneous manifestations in dengue infection. Dendritic cells (Langerhans cells) in the skin may be the early target of infection. It is important to note that these cutaneous presentations along with laboratory tests aid in the early identification of DVI thereby facilitating the timely diagnosis [10].

10.3   Dengue-Induced Skin Rash

Widespread rash or exanthem is estimated to occur in 5–82% of DVI cases [11]. Transient flushing erythema of the face is initial rash which typically appears before or within 24–48 h of onset of symptoms in DVI. Capillary dilatation is considered as predisposing factor underlying the flushing erythema in dengue infection. The second rash manifested as maculopapular or morbilliform eruption and usually occurs 3–6 days after the initiation of fever. Individual lesions may fuse together and give rise to generalized confluent erythema having petechiae and rounded islands of sparing "white islands in a sea of red." This merging of lesions might be attributed to the immune response against virus [12]. However, the rashes during DVI are asymptomatic in majority of cases. Though pruritus is the most troublesome dermal manifestations, its prevalence is lower (16–27%) as compared to other cutaneous presentations [13, 14].

In some patients rashes appear and recover completely, while sometimes they may progress to more generalized eruption [15]. These generalized rashes typically start on the dorsum of the hands and feet and spreads to the arms, legs, and torso. They last for several days and subside without desquamation. Maculopapular or morbilliform rash usually do not appear on palms and soles. The other types of rash may occur but their frequency substantially low [13]. The occurrence of fine macule over pressure areas may accompany the premonitory symptoms and indicates the onset of fever. In some cases, the end of the fever is associated with cutaneous changes such as purpuric eruption on several sites including the buccal cavity, hands, feet, forearms, and legs [15].

10.3.1 Hemorrhagic Manifestations of the Skin

Petechiae, purpura, and ecchymosis are the most common hemorrhagic manifestations on the skin which usually present with positive tourniquet test. These manifestations are more commonly observed in severe forms of DVI (DHF and DSS) and are rarely seen in DF. During Tourniquet test, a blood pressure cuff is used on the upper arm. A pressure to a point midway between systolic and diastolic blood pressures is applied for 5 min. The presence of more than 20 petechiae per 2.5 cm^2 following the application of pressure indicates positive tourniquet test [15]. Hemorrhagic manifestations usually appear 4–5 days following the onset of fever [12].

10.3.2 Differential Diagnosis of Dengue-Induced Skin Rash

The occurrence of rash in febrile patients requires broad differential diagnosis in a broad way. Many viral and bacterial infections are manifested with initial flushing erythema of the chest, head, and neck along with fever at very early stages. Several viral exanthems and bacterial infections are presented with generalized morbilliform eruption in later stages. The infections which may associate with flushing erythema are chikungunya fever, scarlet fever, Kawasaki disease, toxic shock syndrome, and erythema infectiosum (fifth disease parvovirus B-19). Infections associated with morbilliform eruption are measles, rubella, roseola, infectious mononucleosis, secondary syphilis, typhoid fever, chikungunya fever, leptospirosis, acute retroviral syndrome, Rocky Mountain spotted fever, and drug exanthema [4]. The differential diagnosis of DVI is of utmost importance if fever and rash appear in patients residing or returning from dengue-endemic area [15]. Dermatologists may play a vital role in identification of distinctive exanthem of DVI. Since DF can progress to life-threatening severe forms, i.e., DHF/DSS, identification of rash will permit a rapid and early diagnosis of DVI which could be translated into improved disease outcomes among patients. Since rash appears in many other bacterial and viral infections, differentiating features must be considered to optimize the definite diagnosis. Table 10.1 shows varying morphology and distribution of rashes across several infectious diseases.

10.3.3 Pathogenesis of Skin Rash

Dendritic cells of the skin are considered as initial targets of DENV [10]. Currently available data theorize that skin rash results from damaged small blood vessels. However, whether the damage of blood vessels is due to direct destructive effect of DENV or to another cause is still under debate [17]. The pathophysiology of skin rash might be attributed to the interactions between the virus and host cells. Such interactions lead to the release of several chemical mediators which subsequently initiate the immunological mechanisms [18]. The pathologic data indicates

Table 10.1 Differential diagnosis of classic DVI-associated flushing erythema and morbilliform eruption

Disease	Morphology	Distribution of rash	Associated findings
Flushing erythema			
Chikungunya fever	Flushing erythema	Face, upper chest	Severe joint pains, conjunctival injection
Scarlet fever	Membranous desquamation of palms/soles, pinpoint papules on an erythematous background (sand paper), linear petechiae (Pastia's lines)	Generalized, spares palms and soles	Exudative pharyngitis
Kawasaki disease	Desquamation of palms/soles, erythema marginatum, flushing macular erythema, non-pruritic erythematous plaques	Most prominent on trunk and extremities	Conjunctivitis, strawberry tongue, coronary artery aneurysms, lymphadenopathy
Toxic shock syndrome	Erythroderma or scarlatiniform rash	Generalized	Hypotension, renal involvement, focus of infection
Erythema infectiosum (fifth disease parvovirus B-19)	Macular erythema on the face (1–4 days)	Slapped cheek appearance of face followed by extremities, lacy rash over extensor surfaces	Aplastic crisis in sickle cell disease, women may develop arthritis, spontaneous abortions
Morbilliform eruption			
Measles	Erythematous macules and papules, later becomes confluent	Begins on the neck and face, spreads down and become generalized and as it fades it leaves a brownish hue with fine desquamation	Koplik's spots, exudative conjunctivitis, photophobia, pneumonia
German measles (rubella)	Pinpoint maculopapular rash	Begins on the face and spreads to trunk and extremities	Tender cervical lymphadenopathy, transient polyarthralgia and polyarthritis irritability, febrile seizures
Roseola (exanthem subitum HHV-6)	Pale pink macules and papules	Trunk, neck and proximal extremities	Pharyngitis, lymphadenopathy, pinhead petechiae at the junction of soft and hard palate (Forchheimer's spots)

Table 10.1 (continued)

Disease	Morphology	Distribution of rash	Associated findings
Infectious mononucleosis	Polymorphic macular erythema ± petechiae, urticaria, erythema multiforme-like lesions	Generalized	Lymphadenopathy ± condyloma lata ± moth-eaten alopecia
Secondary syphilis	Polymorphic macules/papules/psoriasiform papules	Generalized	Severe joint pains, conjunctival injection
Typhoid fever	2–3 mm pink grouped papules (rose spots) generalized erythema "erythema typhosum"	Generalized, trunk	
Chikungunya fever	Flushing erythema maculopapular lesions, ± petechiae	Trunk and extremities	Severe joint pains, conjunctival injection
Leptospirosis	Morbilliform rash	Generalized	Immune phase: hemorrhage, jaundice, organ failure
Acute retroviral syndrome [16]	Maculopapular rash	Trunk and upper arms ± palms and soles	Myalgia, lymphadenopathy
Rocky mountain spotted fever	Erythematous macules, evolves to petechiae and purpura	Begins on the wrist and ankles; spreads centrally; seen on palms and soles	Hepatosplenomegaly, hyponatremia, myalgias, CNS involvement
Drug exanthem	Maculopapular or urticarial	Generalized symmetric often spares the face and palms and soles may be involved	Periorbital edema, fever

Reference: This table is adapted and modified from reference [12]

superficial perivascular edema, mononuclear infiltration, and endothelial swelling of small blood vessels in dengue patients having skin rash [4]. Immunofluorescence findings have shown DENV antigen, IgM, and complements in the upper dermal plexus of the skin [3]. Based on these findings, the pathophysiology of skin rash may be associated with the reaction of blood vessels to cytokines rather than to widespread viral infection. It can be hypothesized that increased permeability of vessels leads to the expression of inflammatory cell infiltration and dermal edema resulting in skin rash. These findings underscore that blood vessels have high susceptibility for cytokines that are produced by an intact immune system. It must be noted that dengue patients with skin rash have increased itching scores and swelling of palms or soles. However, prolonged disease course or poor prognosis has not been reported in these patients [4].

10.3.4 Prognosis of Dengue-Induced Skin Rash

The prognosis of dengue-induced skin rash is quite satisfactory. Existing literature indicates that DVI patients with skin rash experience itching and swelling of the palms and soles. On the other hand, dengue patients without skin rash have more complications and carry poorer disease outcomes as compared to those with skin rash. The incidence of palm or sole swelling is more profound with morbilliform lesions than with maculopapular or petechial lesions [4].

10.4   Oral Complications in Dengue Infection

The prevalence of oral mucosal complications is approximately 30% in all forms of DVI. However, patients with severe forms of DVI (i.e., DHF, DSS or severe dengue) have higher risks of developing these complications than those with DF [12]. The most prominent oral manifestations include small vesicles on soft palate and erythema or crusting of the tongue and lips. Scleral injection and vesicles on the soft palate have been reported in substantial number of cases [13]. Other mucosal complications may include hemorrhagic bullae on the left lateral surface of the tongue, left sublingual mucous membrane, and on the floor of the mouth. Brown color plagues may appear along with rough surface on the buccal mucosa. Most of the time bleeding can occur when these surfaces are touched. Moreover, spontaneous bleeding from tongue and gingiva (epistaxis) may occur among DVI patients. Nasal bleeding, purpura, petechiae, and ecchymoses are also associated with DVI [19]. The inflammation of the tonsils has also been observed along with hemorrhagic plaques and gum bleeding. Xerostomia (dry mouth) and the tongue coating have also been reported [20].

10.4.1 Dengue-Induced Petechiae

The most common oral manifestation during the course of DVI is petechiae which can be found in the posterior part of the hard palate, soft palate, buccal mucosa, labial mucosa, and tongue. These lesions are reddish-to-purple discoloration caused by leaking of blood from the vessels into the connective tissues. Petechia is a type of purpuric lesions which do not blanch when pressure is applied. Petechia is characterized according to the size of the lesions as petechiae (<0.3 cm), purpura (0.4–0.9 cm), and ecchymosis (>1 cm). Petechiae in combination with gums bleeding, oral ulcer, dryness of mouth, and lip encrusting have been observed in up to 46% of dengue cases [21].

Petechiae are commonly associated with thrombocytopenia as compared to patient with normal platelet count. Thrombocytopenia causes leaking of blood vessels which may result in the formation of petechiae among patients [22]. Thrombocytopenia in DVI is contributed to direct or indirect effect of DENV on bone marrow progenitor cells. DENV inhibits the function of these cells, thus reducing the hematopoietic cell-induced proliferative capacity, resulting in reduced platelets count. Bone marrow hypoplasia can also occur during the acute phase of DVI. The functional disruption of bone marrow progenitor cells is not only associated with reduced platelet counts but may also relate to the deregulation of the plasma kinin system and the immunopathology of DVI. Moreover, DVI affects platelet counts in several other ways including DIC-induced platelet consumption, platelet destruction caused by apoptosis, complement system-related cell lysis, and the production of antiplatelet antibodies [23]. It must be noted that petechiae resolve in same order as they appear with the resolution of other symptoms of dengue.

10.4.2 Dengue-Induced Epistaxis

Bleeding during the course of DVI portends worsening morbidity and sometimes mortality among patients. The toxic hemorrhagic state appears during the 3rd to 5th day of illness following the onset of fever followed by convalescent stage. The most prevalent hemorrhagic manifestations of DIV include epistaxis (gingival bleeding) and skin and gastrointestinal hemorrhages. The pathogenesis of hemorrhage during the course of DVI is multifactorial. Platelet deficiency and dysfunction, vasculopathy, and blood coagulation defects are some important factors contributing to the hemorrhage. DHF-associated thrombocytopenia occurs due to both decreased production and increased destruction of platelets [24, 25]. Epistaxis during dengue is related to thrombocytopenia and may respond well within 48 h of vigorous treatment subjected to the normalization of platelets count [25]. The patients with epistaxis along with other classical symptoms of dengue require prompt referral to the healthcare facility. Since these patients may attend dental clinical at first instance, dentists must thoroughly investigate the cause of bleeding, and suspected dengue cases must be referred for timely management. The oral complications during the course of DVI urge the role of dentists and dermatologists in dengue control programs. Appropriately structured educational programs for these professionals could be translated into timely referral of patients which will further reduce the diagnostic delay of dengue.

10.5   Dengue-Induced Intracranial Hemorrhage

Dengue-induced intracranial hemorrhage (ICH) has been observed in isolated case reports. Many of these cases have bleeding even in the absence of any predisposing factor for intracranial bleeding [26, 27]. Moreover, existing data also indicate that intracranial bleeding may occur even in the absence of bleeding from any other site. Microcapillary hemorrhage during the course of DVI causes intracranial bleeding, cerebral edema, hyponatremia, cerebral anoxia, and release of toxic products [27]. The pathogenesis of dengue-associated ICH is not clear. However, several factors contribute towards this serious and life-threatening intricacy. It is hypothesized that mild form of DIC, prolonged prothrombin time, thrombocytopenia, and hepatic anomalies contribute synergistically to dengue-induced ICH [16]. Deranged prothrombin time substantially associates with intracranial bleeding in dengue. However, there are many other factors which alone or in combination with each other may precipitate bleeding intricacies. These include platelet count of less than 50,000/mm^3, biphasic pattern of fever, elevated liver transaminases (particularly ALT), and hemoconcentration [26, 28]. The documented evidence suggests that DENV can cause the breakdown of blood–brain and cerebrospinal fluid barriers during its clinical course [29]. It is interesting to note that macrophage migration inhibitory factor (MIF) is produced in dengue infection. MIF may contribute to vascular hyperpermeability and hemostatic abnormalities. Therefore, the blocking of MIF may be an effective measure to prevent the dengue-associated hemorrhages [30]. For dengue patients with headache or alteration in mental status, intracerebral hemorrhage should be highly suspected. Available information demonstrates that hemorrhage within the tumor of the pituitary gland resulting in pituitary apoplexy can also occur in dengue patients [31].

The causative factors of ICH such as vasculopathy and platelet dysfunction are usually present and irreversible even after the surgery. Therefore, dengue-associated intracranial bleeding is inherently harder to manage [32]. Surgery and optimal medical management are considered primary therapeutic options for all types of intracranial hemorrhage. Since dengue-induced intracranial bleeding is rare, it will be too early to advocate if these patients should be treated like any other spontaneous ICH. Moreover, advantages of surgery over medical treatment and timing to perform surgical interventions are two questions without any satisfactory answers. Existing evidences suggest improved outcome if surgery is performed within 8 h of hemorrhage [33, 34]. However, available data from case series on dengue-induced intracranial hemorrhage suggest supportive therapy as mainstay of treatment. The need of platelet transfusions is rare during the management of dengue. However, platelets can be infused to patients with substantial drop of platelet counts or those with significant bleeding. The recommendation of transfusion is based on the levels of platelet. Platelets below 20,000/mL without hemorrhage or approximately 50,000/mL with hemorrhage are indicators of transfusion in many cases. Surgical interventions can also be applied for ocular and intracranial complications. However, correction of coagulation defect with platelet count above 100,000/mL should be considered before commencing the surgical procedures [26, 27, 34, 35]. Though dengue-induced intracranial hemorrhage is infrequent, little is known about its management, treatment modalities, and diagnosis. Further studies are needed to ascertain the relationship of dengue with intracranial bleeding along with its diagnostic and treatment differences from intracranial bleeding of other causes.

10.6   Dengue-Induced Thyroiditis

The involvement of thyroid glands during the clinical course of DVI is rarely reported. Recent investigations underscore subacute thyroiditis as a potential complication of expanded dengue syndrome [36, 37]. Clinical manifestations of subacute thyroiditis include pain or discomfort in the neck region, tender diffuse goiter, and a predictable course of thyroid function evolution. Hyperthyroidism is a typical presentation of thyroid impairments which follow euthyroidism, hypothyroidism, and ultimately restoration of normal thyroid function. Both direct action of viruses and post-viral inflammatory processes contribute to the development of subacute thyroiditis. Onset of thyroiditis is observed in majority of patients having a history of (typically 2–8 weeks beforehand) upper respiratory tract infection. There have been many reports indicating the association between thyroiditis with measles, mumps, coxsackievirus, adenovirus and many other viral infections [38]. Dengue-induced thyroiditis might be attributed to the direct infection or post-infectious immune injury during the course of DVI. Many times thyroiditis goes unnoticed because it mimics pharyngitis, but thyroid swelling with pain, fever, and features of thyrotoxicosis is a classical symptom of dengue infection. The pain during thyroid swelling may even radiate to the ear [39]. Thyroid crisis or thyroid storm has also been reported in association with the occurrence of DVI. Thyroid storm can be aggravated during the course of dengue fever especially in patients who present with undiagnosed hyperthyroidism [40, 41]. Concomitant appearance of acute transverse myelitis and subacute thyroiditis has been reported in the literature [36].

The promising treatment of subacute thyroiditis is currently not available owing to the lack of clinical trials. Patients can be treated with aspirin, a nonsteroidal anti-inflammatory drug (e.g., ibuprofen) or prednisolone [38]. The symptoms of hyperthyroidism occur infrequently, and if present, then they are mild and short-lived in nature, thereby therapy for hyperthyroidism is often not necessary in majority of the patients. However, symptoms of hyperthyroidism can be bothersome and may be treated with the use of beta blockers. Since aspirin and few NSAIDs are associated with high bleeding risks particularly in the presence of thrombocytopenia and frontal lobe hematoma, oral prednisolone can be a preferred choice to treat the acute inflammation [37].

10.7   Dengue-Induced Splenial Lesion Syndrome

Splenium is one of the anatomical divisions of corpus callosum, the largest fiber bundle which connects the cerebral cortex of the left and right cerebral hemispheres. Other anatomical divisions of corpus callosum include rostrum, genu, and body. Corpus callosum promotes the functional integration of sensory and motor functions. All four anatomical divisions play a pivotal role in relaying sensory, motor, and cognitive information from homologous regions in the two cerebral hemispheres. Owing to the rich blood supply from three main arterial systems (the anterior communicating artery, the pericallosal artery, and the posterior pericallosal artery), infarctions of the corpus callosum are infrequent [42]. Reversible splenial lesion syndrome (RESLES) has been reported during the course of DVI in the presence of pre-existing encephalopathy [43–45].

RESLES has both infectious and non-infectious causes. The syndrome is also termed as mild encephalitis with reversible splenial lesion [31] in case of infectious cause. Some authors have also proposed the name "cytotoxic lesions of the corpus callosum (CLOCCs)" due to the pathophysiological mechanisms [46]. RESLES frequently occurs in infectious encephalopathy due to influenza virus, rotavirus, measles, herpes virus, adenovirus, mumps, Epstein-Barr virus, and *Escherichia coli* [42]. Non-infectious causes include metabolic disorders such as hypoglycemia and hypernatremia, high-altitude cerebral edema (HACE), and antiepileptic drug withdrawal [47–50].

Clinical manifestations of RESLES are nonspecific, prodromal, and complex. Most of the patients present with gait disorders, apraxia, agraphia, tactile anomia, and alien hand syndrome [47]. Diagnostic findings from MRI suggest the neuroimaging appearance of a round-shaped, non-enhancing lesion centered in the splenium of the corpus callosum. However, these lesions resolve after a variable duration [42]. Diffusion tensor imaging (DTI) is another tool to understand the microstructural white matter tract changes associated with Mild encephalitis/encephalopathy with reversible splenial lesion (MERS) [45].

The pathogenesis of RESLES or MERS during the course of DVI is not clear. It is hypothesized that increased endothelium permeability and hypo-sodium during DVI induces MERS among patients [44]. Another study suggests vascular distribution, direct viral invasion, and arginine vasopressin suppression as major contributors of MERS in dengue infection [45]. However, further studies are recommended to illustrate a causal relationship between DVI and MERS.

Patients with dengue-associated MERS or RESLES should be managed conservatively with supportive fluid rehydration. These patients show satisfactory clinical recovery within few days of illness with complete normalization of blood count. However, serial MRI and DTI should be planned through appropriate follow-up in order to ascertain the long-term outcomes [43, 45].

10.8   Dengue-Induced Hemophagocytic Lymphohistiocytosis

Hemophagocytic lymphohistiocytosis (HLH) is a rare but potentially fatal hematologic disorder. It is clinically manifested as hyperinflammation, prolonged fever, jaundice, uncontrolled proliferation of activated lymphocytes, pancytopenia, and hepatosplenomegaly [51]. Both primary (familial) and secondary (acquired) etiologies contribute to HLH. Most of the cases with familial HLH are caused by mutation in five genes which usually occur within the first 2 years of life. Secondary HLH is more common than primary and caused by strong immunological activation associated with autoimmune disorders, malignancies, or infections. The most common cause of infectious HLH is Epstein-Barr virus (EBV). Other infections associated with HLH are tuberculosis, HIV, cytomegalovirus, and parvovirus B19 [52]. Treatment of both primary and secondary HLH differs due to underlying pathogenesis. Familial HLH is fatal if timely treatment is not provided. Its treatment includes hematopoietic stem cell transplantation which replaces defective immune effector cells. Secondary HLH can be effectively managed with high-dose cortico-steroids, intravenous immunoglobulin (IVIG), and cyclosporine. Sometimes cyclosporine is given with etoposide to dampen the immune response [51–53].

Dengue-induced HLH is more common in children as compared to adults. Moreover, severe forms of DVI such as DHF and DSS portend substantial risks of development of HLH. DENV causes infection of T cells resulting in cytokine production leading to uncontrolled histiocytic activity. It has been hypothesized that the increased production of cytokines, interferon-γ, and tumor necrosis factor-α (TNF-α) plays vital role in the pathogenesis of HLH during the course of DVI. Out of four recognized serotypes of dengue viruses, only three have been attributed to cause HLH (DEN1, DEN3, and DEN4) [54–56]. HLH is usually diagnosed in the second week of illness in most of the dengue cases [57].

Dengue-associated HLH may progress to infection-associated hemophagocytic syndrome (IAHS), a highly fatal complication. Early identification and initiation of steroidal therapy would be of paramount importance for the successful management of DVI complicated by HLH. Since DVI and HLH share several common signs and symptoms (fever, hepatosplenomegaly, leukopenia, and thrombocytopenia), the condition remains underrecognized in the majority of cases. There is a dire need to investigate the DENV as a potential trigger for IAHS [58].

References

1. Rathore AP, St. John AL. Immune responses to dengue virus in the skin. Open Biol. 2018;8(8):180087.
2. Marchette N, Halstead S, Falkler W Jr, Stenhouse A, Nash D. Studies on the pathogenesis of dengue infection in monkeys. III. Sequential distribution of virus in primary and heterologous infections. J Infect Dis. 1973;128(1):23–30.
3. de Anorno R, Botet M, Gubler SD, Duane J, Garcia C, Laboy E, Espada F, et al. The absence of dengue virus in the skin lesions of dengue fever. Int J Dermatol. 1985;24(1):48–51.
4. Huang H-W, Tseng H-C, Lee C-H, Chuang H-Y, Lin S-H. Clinical significance of skin rash in dengue fever: a focus on discomfort, complications, and disease outcome. Asian Pac J Trop Med. 2016;9(7):713–8.
5. Le Duyen HT, Cerny D, Trung DT, Pang J, Velumani S, Toh YX, et al. Skin dendritic cell and T cell activation associated with dengue shock syndrome. Sci Rep. 2017;7(1):14224.
6. Schmid MA, Harris E. Monocyte recruitment to the dermis and differentiation to dendritic cells increases the targets for dengue virus replication. PLoS Pathog. 2014;10(12):e1004541.
7. Cerny D, Haniffa M, Shin A, Bigliardi P, Tan BK, Lee B, et al. Selective susceptibility of human skin antigen presenting cells to productive dengue virus infection. PLoS Pathog. 2014;10(12):e1004548.
8. Diamond MS, Edgil D, Roberts TG, Lu B, Harris E. Infection of human cells by dengue virus is modulated by different cell types and viral strains. J Virol. 2000;74(17):7814–23.

9. Mahboob A, Iqbal Z, Javed R, Taj A, Munir A, Saleemi MA, et al. Dermatological manifestations of dengue fever. J Ayub Med Coll Abbottabad. 2012;24(1):52–4.

10. Wu S-JL, Grouard-Vogel G, Sun W, Mascola JR, Brachtel E, Putvatana R, et al. Human skin Langerhans cells are targets of dengue virus infection. Nat Med. 2000;6(7):816.

11. Itoda I, Masuda G, Suganuma A, Imamura A, Ajisawa A, Yamada K-I, et al. Clinical features of 62 imported cases of dengue fever in Japan. Am J Trop Med Hyg. 2006;75(3):470–4.

12. Thomas EA, John M, Kanish B. Mucocutaneous manifestations of dengue fever. Indian J Dermatol. 2010;55(1):79.

13. Chadwick D, Arch B, Wilder-Smith A, Paton N. Distinguishing dengue fever from other infections on the basis of simple clinical and laboratory features: application of logistic regression analysis. J Clin Virol. 2006;35(2):147–53.

14. Thomas EA, John M, Bhatia A. Cutaneous manifestations of dengue viral infection in Punjab (North India). Int J Dermatol. 2007;46(7):715–9.

15. Pincus LB, Grossman ME, Fox LP. The exanthem of dengue fever: clinical features of two US tourists traveling abroad. J Am Acad Dermatol. 2008;58(2):308–16.

16. Shivbalan S, Anandnathan K, Balasubramanian S, Datta M, Amalraj E. Predictors of spontaneous bleeding in dengue. Indian J Pediatr. 2004;71(1):33–6.

17. Mims C. Pathogenesis of rashes in virus diseases. Bacteriol Rev. 1966;30(4):739.

18. Teixeira MG, Barreto ML. Diagnosis and management of dengue. BMJ. 2009;339:b4338.

19. Byatnal A, Mahajan N, Koppal S, Ravikiran A, Thriveni R, Parvathi Devi M. Unusual yet isolated oral manifestations of persistent thrombocytopenia: a rare case report. Braz J Oral Sci. 2013;12(3):233–6.

20. Mithra R, Baskaran P, Sathyakumar M. Oral presentation in dengue hemorrhagic fever: a rare entity. J Nat Sci Biol Med. 2013;4(1):264.

21. Govindaraj S, Jayaraman R, Daniel MJ, Subbiah S, Vasudevan SS, Kumaran JV. Oral manifestations of dengue fever. Sahel Med J. 2018;21(4):194.

22. de Lima AAS, de Oliveira Melo NSF, Gil FBD. Oral manifestation of thrombocytopenia in immunosuppressed patient—report of case. J Oral Diag. 2016;1(1):1.

23. de Azeredo EL, Monteiro RQ, de Oliveira Pinto LM. Thrombocytopenia in dengue: interrelationship between virus and the imbalance between coagulation and fibrinolysis and inflammatory mediators. Mediat Inflamm. 2015;2015:313842.

24. Chiu Y-C, Wu K-L, Kuo C-H, Hu T-H, Chou Y-P, Chuah S-K, et al. Endoscopic findings and management of dengue patients with upper gastrointestinal bleeding. Am J Trop Med Hyg. 2005;73(2):441–4.

25. Khan S, Gupta N, Maheshwari S. Acute gingival bleeding as a complication of dengue hemorrhagic fever. J Indian Soc Periodontol. 2013;17(4):520.

26. Sam JE, Gee TS, Nasser AW. Deadly intracranial bleed in patients with dengue fever: a series of nine patients and review of literature. J Neurosci Rural Pract. 2016;7(3):423.

27. Kumar R, Prakash O, Sharma B. Intracranial hemorrhage in dengue fever: management and outcome: a series of 5 cases and review of literature. Surg Neurol. 2009;72(4):429–33.

28. Rajapakse S, de Silva NL, Weeratunga P, Rodrigo C, Fernando SD. Prophylactic and therapeutic interventions for bleeding in dengue: a systematic review. Trans R Soc Trop Med Hyg. 2017;111(10):433–9.

29. Puccioni-Sohler M, Rosadas C, Cabral-Castro MJ. Neurological complications in dengue infection: a review for clinical practice. Arq Neuropsiquiatr. 2013;71(9B):667–71.

30. Chuang Y-C, Chen H-R, Yeh T-M. Pathogenic roles of macrophage migration inhibitory factor during dengue virus infection. Mediat Inflamm. 2015;2015:1.

31. Wildemberg L, Neto L, Niemeyer P, Gasparetto E, Chimelli L, Gadelha M. Association of dengue hemorrhagic fever with multiple risk factors for pituitary apoplexy. Endocr Pract. 2012;18(5):e97–e101.

32. Morgenstern LB, Hemphill JC III, Anderson C, Becker K, Broderick JP, Connolly ES Jr, et al. Guidelines for the management of spontaneous intracerebral hemorrhage: a guideline for healthcare professionals from the American Heart Association/American Stroke Association. Stroke. 2010;41(9):2108–29.

33. Mendelow AD, Gregson BA, Rowan EN, Murray GD, Gholkar A, Mitchell PM, et al. Early surgery versus initial conservative treatment in patients with spontaneous supratentorial lobar intracerebral haematomas (STICH II): a randomised trial. Lancet. 2013;382(9890):397–408.

34. Gregson BA, Broderick JP, Auer LM, Batjer H, Chen X-C, Juvela S, et al. Individual patient data subgroup meta-analysis of surgery for spontaneous supratentorial intracerebral hemorrhage. Stroke. 2012;43(6):1496–504.

35. Ali N, Usman M, Syed N, Khurshid M. Haemorrhagic manifestations and utility of haematological parameters in dengue fever: a tertiary care centre experience at Karachi. Scand J Infect Dis. 2007;39(11–12):1025–8.

36. Mo Z, Dong Y, Chen X, Yao H, Zhang B. Acute transverse myelitis and subacute thyroiditis associated with dengue viral infection: a case report and literature review. Exp Ther Med. 2016;12(4):2331–5.

37. Assir MZK, Jawa A, Ahmed HI. Expanded dengue syndrome: subacute thyroiditis and intracerebral hemorrhage. BMC Infect Dis. 2012;12(1):240.

38. Samuels MH. Subacute, silent, and postpartum thyroiditis. Med Clin. 2012;96(2):223–33.

39. Bhushan D. Subacute thyroiditis: a rare complication of dengue. J Assoc Physicians India. 2018;66(6):112.

40. Dwipayana IMP, Nugraha IA, Semadi S, Wirawan IMS. Thyroid crisis in a toxic multinodular goiter patient triggered by a DEN-3 subtype dengue infection. Biomed Pharmacol J. 2017;10(3):1293–300.

41. Chong HW, See KC, Phua J. Thyroid storm with multiorgan failure. Thyroid. 2010;20(3):333–6.

42. Zhu Y, Zheng J, Zhang L, Zeng Z, Zhu M, Li X, et al. Reversible splenial lesion syndrome associated with encephalitis/encephalopathy presenting with great clinical heterogeneity. BMC Neurol. 2016;16(1):49.

43. Sathananthasarma P, Weeratunga PN, Chang T. Reversible splenial lesion syndrome associated with dengue fever: a case report. BMC Res Notes. 2018;11(1):412.

44. Saito N, Kitashouji E, Kojiro M, Furumoto A, Morimoto K, Morita K, et al. A case of clinically mild encephalitis/encephalopathy with a reversible splenial lesion due to dengue fever. Kansenshogaku Zasshi. 2015;89(4):465–9.

45. Fong CY, Khine MMK, Peter AB, Lim WK, Rozalli FI, Rahmat K. Mild encephalitis/encephalopathy with reversible splenial lesion (MERS) due to dengue virus. J Clin Neurosci. 2017;36:73–5.

46. Starkey J, Kobayashi N, Numaguchi Y, Moritani T. Cytotoxic lesions of the corpus callosum that show restricted diffusion: mechanisms, causes, and manifestations. Radiographics. 2017;37(2):562–76.

47. Yang L-L, Huang Y-N, Cui Z-T. Clinical features of acute corpus callosum infarction patients. Int J Clin Exp Pathol. 2014;7(8):5160.

48. Bulakbasi N, Kocaoglu M, Tayfun C, Ucoz T. Transient splenial lesion of the corpus callosum in clinically mild influenza-associated encephalitis/encephalopathy. Am J Neuroradiol. 2006;27(9):1983–6.

49. Garcia-Monco JC, Cortina IE, Ferreira E, Martínez A, Ruiz L, Cabrera A, et al. Reversible splenial lesion syndrome (RESLES): what's in a name? J Neuroimaging. 2011;21(2):e1–e14.

50. Jeong TO, Yoon JC, Lee JB, Jin YH, Hwang SB. Reversible splenial lesion syndrome (RESLES) following glufosinate ammonium poisoning. J Neuroimaging. 2015;25(6):1050–2.

51. Janka GE. Familial and acquired hemophagocytic lymphohistiocytosis. Eur J Pediatr. 2007;166(2):95–109.

52. Fisman DN. Hemophagocytic syndromes and infection. Emerg Infect Dis. 2000;6(6):601.

53. Niece JA, Rogers ZR, Ahmad N, Langevin AM, McClain KL. Hemophagocytic lymphohistiocytosis in Texas: observations on ethnicity and race. Pediatr Blood Cancer. 2010;54(3):424–8.

54. Khurram M, Faheem M, Umar M, Yasin A, Qayyum W, Ashraf A, et al. Hemophagocytic lymphohistiocytosis complicating dengue and *Plasmodium vivax* coinfection. Case Rep Med. 2015;2015:1.

55. Nakamura I, Nakamura-Uchiyama F, Komiya N, Ohnishi K. A case of dengue fever with viral-associated hemophagocytic syndrome. Kansenshogaku Zasshi. 2009;83(1):60–3.
56. Ellis EM, Pérez-Padilla J, González L, Lebo E, Baker C, Sharp T, et al. Unusual cluster in time and space of dengue-associated hemophagocytic lymphohistiocytosis in Puerto Rico. Washington, DC: American Society of Hematology; 2013.
57. Koshy M, Mishra AK, Agrawal B, Kurup AR, Hansdak SG. Dengue fever complicated by hemophagocytosis. Oxf Med Case Reports. 2016;2016(6):121–4.
58. Chung SM, Song JY, Kim W, Choi MJ, Jeon JH, Kang S, et al. Dengue-associated hemophagocyticlymphohistiocytosis in an adult: a case report and literature review. Medicine. 2017;96(8):e6159.

Conclusions and Suggestions

11

11.1 Conclusions

The evolution of dengue viral infection (DVI) from breakbone fever or dandy fever to expanded dengue syndrome (EDS) takes more than 20 years. The World Health Organization (WHO) played a momentous role in curbing the growing encumbrance of disease due to vast geographical spread of dengue virus (DENV). Dengue was classified as differentiated and undifferentiated infection according to the WHO 1997 guidelines. The differentiated patients were further grouped into classical dengue and dengue hemorrhagic fever (DHF) based on the levels of platelets and hematocrit. The DHF of grade 3 and 4 was classified as dengue shock syndrome (DSS) in these guidelines [1]. However, due to several diagnostic and management confusions, WHO revised its classification in 2009 with emphasis on the presence of warning signs among patients. According to this new classification, DVI can be classified into probable dengue, dengue with warning signs, dengue without warning signs, and severe dengue [2]. The last modification that WHO did in dengue guidelines was incorporating the term "EDS" or "atypical complications" for diagnosis due to increasing number of reports related to organ involvements during the course of DVI [3].

Dengue-associated mortality is less than 1% but may exceed to 20% in untreated cases. Mortality during the course of DVI is primarily linked to the associated complications. Dengue viral infection classically presents with sharply dropping platelet counts, which may or may not be associated with plasma leakage. The plasma leakage during the course of DVI may progress to either compensated or uncompensated shock. Since shock syndrome results in reduced cellular perfusions and disturbed hemodynamic stability, patients develop multi-organ failure or disturbance during the course of infection. Dengue infection with failure of two or more organs is accompanied by high mortality. Apart from the classical presentation, dengue infection can result in a myriad of unusual clinical manifestations, which are grouped under the title "expanded dengue syndrome (EDS)." The term of EDS is first time coined by the World Health Organization (WHO) in its guidelines on the

© Springer Nature Singapore Pte Ltd. 2021
T. H. Mallhi et al., *Expanded Dengue Syndrome*,
https://doi.org/10.1007/978-981-15-7337-8_11

management of dengue infection [3]. EDS primarily appears among patients with hematological presentations such as DHF, DSS or severe dengue. However, the prevalence of EDS among dengue patients without any evidence of plasma leakage is also prominent in the literature [4].

Initially dengue infection was considered a viral disease with hematological anomalies. With the recent advancements in research and due to growing body of evidences on dengue-associated atypical manifestations, DVI emerged as a complex collection of symptoms rather than a single entity. Considering all the chapters of the current book, it is clearly understood that dengue virus affects almost every organ system of the patients. These findings instigate the dire need of multidisciplinary management of dengue patients. Clinicians from varying disciplines should be aware of these intricacies, particularly in areas where dengue is hyperendemic or endemic. In most of the cases, these complications are either under-reported or remain unrecognized, particularly during the dengue epidemics when hospital staff and resources are limited to tackle the increasing number of patients. It must be noted that these complications can be prevented with timely diagnosis and judiciary management [5].

Of these atypical complications accompanied by dengue infection, neurological, hepatic, and cardiac involvements frequently occur among patients and are accompanied by increased morbidity and mortality [6]. These manifestations do not only pose substantial encumbrance to patient but also carry increased burden to healthcare system in terms of cost of care. Recently, kidneys evolve as the major organ affected by dengue virus through several pathological mechanisms resulting in acute kidney injury (AKI) or glomerulonephritis. Dengue-related AKI is found to be associated with high morbidity, mortality, and unsatisfactory recovery of renal profile among patients [7–9]. With the increasing burden of DVI globally, neurological complications are increasingly being recognized among patients. Neurological involvements during the course of DVI are life-threatening; thus, disease prevention and early recognition of any unusual manifestations are only available options [10].

Despite growing body of evidences in the literature, EDS is still under-recognized and under-reported during the course of DVI. Physicians with updated knowledge and high degree of suspicion can identify the EDS in timely manners and can take appropriate measures. It has been well documented that any diagnostic delay may lead to worsening of clinical conditions. Timely identification and early response to atypical manifestations can not only prevent deteriorating complications but may also avoid unnecessary procedures [11].

It has been observed that EDS is multisystemic and multifacetal in nature. The association of disease severity and patient's demographics with the development and severity of atypical manifestations is not clearly understood. Existing literature demonstrates disparity regarding any relationship of dengue virus and patient's characteristics with EDS. These findings urge more focused and comprehensive investigations to explore such relationships so that high-risk patients could be identified immediately during their presentation to the hospitals. This book attempted to include all reported complications of DVI available in the literature till date. The summary of these complications are described in Table 11.1.

Table 11.1 Expanded dengue syndrome in nutshell

Organ system	Complications
Gastrohepatic	Elevated transaminases
	Acute liver failure
	Transaminitis
	Gastrointestinal bleeding
	Intestinal perforation
	Pancreatitis
Renal	Acute kidney injury (previously known as "acute renal failure")
	Glomerulonephritis
	Nephrotic syndrome
	Hematuria
	Electrolyte disturbances
	Acute exacerbations of "chronic kidney disease"
	Chronic elevation of serum creatinine
Cardiac	Myocarditis
	ECG abnormalities
Respiratory	Acute respiratory distress syndrome
	Pleural effusion
	Respiratory failure
	Diffuse alveolar hemorrhage
Neurological	Encephalopathy
	Encephalitis
	Meningitis
	Myositis
	Myelitis
	Acute disseminated encephalomyelitis
	Neuromyelitis optica
	Optic neuritis
	Post-infectious encephalopathy
	Guillain-Barré syndrome
	Neuritis brachialis
Musculoskeletal	Rhabdomyolysis
	Myalgia
	Myositis
	Osteonecrosis of the jaw
	Hypokalemic paralysis
	Post-infection fatigue syndrome
	Myasthenia gravis
	Arthralgia
	Sacroiliitis
	Bone marrow suppression
Lymphoreticular	Splenic rupture
	Lymphadenopathy
	Splenomegaly
	Lymph node infarction

(continued)

Table 11.1 (continued)

Organ system	Complications
Ophthalmic	*Complications of anterior segment of the eye*
	Subconjunctival hemorrhage
	Anterior uveitis
	Intermediate uveitis
	Shallow anterior chamber
	Ciliary congestion
	Keratitis
	Corneal erosion
	Acute angle closure
	Complications of posterior segment of the eye
	Maculopathy
	Macular edema
	Vitreous hemorrhage
	Vascular occlusions (vein occlusions)
	Arterial occlusion of the superotemporal macular branch
	Retinal hemorrhages
	Posterior uveitis
	Foveolitis
	Serous retinal detachment
	Neuro-ophthalmic disorders
	Optic neuritis
	Cranial nerve palsies
	Neuromyelitis optica
	Miscellaneous ophthalmic complications
	Panophthalmitis
	Periorbital ecchymosis
Miscellaneous	Exanthema
	Petechiae
	Epistaxis
	Intracranial hemorrhage
	Thyroiditis
	Splenial lesion syndrome
	Hemophagocytic lymphohistiocytosis

11.2 Suggestions and Recommendations for Healthcare Professionals

Keeping in view the increasing burden of EDS, the following suggestions would be of paramount importance to curb the growing encumbrance of these atypical manifestations:

- Public awareness seminars on the importance of timely reporting to the hospitals, as diagnostic delay may lead to development of EDS among patients
- Workshops and educational seminar series on expanded dengue syndrome for healthcare professionals, particularly for those dealing with dengue patients

- Identification of high-risk patients with increased propensity of developing EDS
- Development of sensitive and specific predictive models for risk assessment of any atypical manifestations during the DVI
- Implementation of multidisciplinary approach in patient's management
- Development of rapid reporting and call or alert system for other healthcare professionals once any unusual manifestation is suspected
- Design and implementation of treatment algorithm or protocols for the management of EDS
- Multidisciplinary approach in decision-making
- Development of decision-making algorithms for treating and referring any unusual complications
- Follow-up of patients recovering from any atypical condition to ascertain the long-term sequel
- Consideration of high-risk patients to be treated under intensive care
- Documentation of EDS cases along with management and follow-up data
- Multidisciplinary research on EDS
- Incorporation of EDS management in dengue treatment guidelines
- Inclusion of EDS in graduation curriculum
- Design and conduction of research studies to evaluate the knowledge of healthcare professionals towards EDS

A large number of studies report the atypical manifestations in dengue patients. However, these studies are accompanied by several shortcomings which preclude practitioners to draw firm conclusions in real-world setting. Most of the studies on EDS are uncontrolled which are either case reports or case series conducted on a limited number of patients. Moreover, there are wide variations in definitions and diagnostic criteria used in the literature, making it difficult or sometimes impossible to compare the findings across studies. Moreover, there is no evidence-based literature available which could be used in decision-making on EDS. The World Health Organization (WHO) can play an important role in strengthening the research by providing uniform methodologies for epidemiological studies. Development and implementation of reporting tools will boost the research uniformity around the globe. There are also dearth of investigations ascertaining the high-risk patients of EDS and decision-making factors. In addition, disparity in the classification of dengue infection is another barrier to unanimity of research methodology.

References

1. Khursheed M, Khan UR, Ejaz K, Fayyaz J, Qamar I, Razzak J. A comparison of WHO guidelines issued in 1997 and 2009 for dengue fever-single centre experience. J Pak Med Assoc. 2013;63(6):670.
2. World Health Organization, Special Programme for Research and Training in Tropical Diseases, World Health Organization. Department of Control of Neglected Tropical Diseases, World Health Organization. Epidemic and Pandemic Alert and Response. Dengue: guidelines for diagnosis, treatment, prevention and control. Geneva: World Health Organization; 2009.

3. WHO-SEARO. Comprehensive guidelines for prevention and control of dengue and dengue hemorrhagic fever. Geneva: World Health Organization; 2011.
4. Islam QT, Hossain HT, Khandaker MA, Ahasan HN, Majumder M, Jabeen T. Dengue expanded syndrome: an unusual presentation. Bangladesh J Med. 2018;29(1):45–7.
5. Kadam D, Salvi S, Chandanwale A. Expanded dengue. J Assoc Physicians India. 2016;64(7):59–63.
6. Gulati S, Maheshwari A. Atypical manifestations of dengue. Tropical Med Int Health. 2007;12(9):1087–95.
7. Mallhi TH, Khan AH, Adnan AS, Sarriff A, Khan YH, Gan SH. Short-term renal outcomes following acute kidney injury among dengue patients: a follow-up analysis from large prospective cohort. PLoS One. 2018;13(2):e0192510.
8. Mallhi TH, Sarriff A, Adnan AS, Khan YH, Hamzah AA, Jummaat F, et al. Dengue-induced acute kidney injury (DAKI): a neglected and fatal complication of dengue viral infection-a systematic review. J Coll Physicians Surg Pak. 2015;25(11):828–34.
9. Mallhi TH, Khan AH, Adnan AS, Sarriff A, Khan YH, Jummaat F. Incidence, characteristics and risk factors of acute kidney injury among dengue patients: a retrospective analysis. PLoS One. 2015;10:9.
10. Kumar A, Margekar SL. Neurological manifestations in dengue. Indian J Med Spec. 2016;7(4):152–4.
11. Anam AM, Shumy F, Rabbani R, Polash MMI, Huq S, Shareef A. Expanded dengue syndrome: gastrointestinal manifestations. Bangladesh Crit Care J. 2018;6:34–9.